Managerial Innovation in the Metropolitan Hospital

Dalton E. McFarland

MANAGERIAL INNOVATION IN THE METROPOLITAN HOSPITAL

PRAEGER

PRAEGER SPECIAL STUDIES • PRAEGER SCIENTIFIC

Library of Congress Cataloging in Publication Data

McFarland, Dalton E
   Managerial innovation in the metropolitan hospital.

   Bibliography: p.
   Includes index.
   1. Hospitals--Administration--Case studies.
2. Organizational change--Case studies. I. Title.
[DNLM: 1. Hospital administration. WX150.3 M143m]
RA971.M246   658'.91'36211   79-14551
ISBN 0-03-051341-3

Published in 1979 by Praeger Publishers
A Division of Holt, Rinehart and Winston/CBS, Inc.
383 Madison Avenue, New York, New York 10017 U.S.A.

© 1979 by Praeger Publishers

Printed in the United States of America

With appreciation to

William Foote Whyte
Teacher, Researcher, Humanist

———————————————————————

Research is a high-hat word

that scares a lot of people.

It needn't. It is rather simple.

Essentially research is

nothing but a state of mind—

a friendly, welcoming attitude

toward change—

— Charles F. Kettering

PREFACE

The purpose of this book is to provide an integrated management analysis of the themes of innovation and change as reflected in the work of key administrators and managers in the large metropolitan hospital. This is a timely theme since hospitals today play a central role in a health care system, undergoing the stress and strain of turbulent social, political, and economic problems.

This exploratory study is part of a long-run series of investigations of the processes of innovation and change in health care organizations generally and of the interplay of our major social institutions and their organizational components. The primary source of the data analyzed in this study consisted of observations and interviews in a large metropolitan acute care private hospital. The field study methods utilized were those of applied anthropology and sociology. Seventy-two depth interviews provided the source materials; 54 of these were in the primary site and an additional 18 were obtained from top administrators in hospitals and health care organizations located in the same metropolitan area as the main site. This field work began in late 1973 and was completed in late 1977.

A conceptual model is introduced as a framework for analyzing the findings reported here. The model brings together the key elements of the process of managerial innovation and change, so that they may be examined as management phenomena. Within this framework, the interview data are extensively reported in the informants' own words, so that the reader may vicariously experience their feelings and attitudes. The model systematically organizes concepts of innovation and change that are usually treated in an ad hoc, fragmented fashion.

I make no apology for the fact that this is essentially a case study, and that the methods employed are qualitative rather than statistical. The hospital is a prototypical organization of health care services, and few comprehensive, analytical case studies of total hospital organizations are available to explain it. At the same time, I acknowledge the limitations that case studies present as to the generalizations the findings permit. I believe these limitations are offset by the need to penetrate more deeply into the recesses of ongoing concrete situations, so that propositions and hypotheses may be derived for later examination by other methods.

This book is intended for the use of administrators, public officials, trustees, teachers, consultants, people in allied health care, students, researchers, technicians, and other professionals whose concern for the improvement of hospital management come together in the sharing of their work and responsibility, if not of their points of view.

The names of all organizations and the names and titles of all persons in this study have been changed to preserve their anonymity. However, I am grateful to the participating hospital administrators and staff members (who must go unnamed) for their time and cooperation. I deeply appreciate the capable work of colleagues and associates who assisted me in this project. Three research assistants at the University of Alabama in Birmingham helped me with enthusiasm and imagination. Mr. David Naler and Miss Carolyn O'Donnell conducted many of the interviews. Miss O'Donnell coded and helped analyze the enormous volume of interview data. Mrs. Michael Neilson ably assisted in checking references, proofreading, and in many other essential tasks. To Miss Marcia Stokes and Miss Robbie Armstrong I express my thanks for patiently typing and retyping the project materials and this manuscript. I wish also to offer my thanks to the University of Alabama in Birmingham for funding this project through three annual research grants from the University College Faculty Research Fund, and to Dean M. Gene Newport and Professor W. Jack Duncan of the School of Business for their encouragement and unfailing support. I am also grateful to my colleagues throughout the university, particularly those in the School of Business, School of Nursing, and the School of Community and Allied Health. They provided an inspiring and sustaining community of discourse from which I profited without measure. I am also deeply indebted to my wife, Jean A. McFarland, for her enlightened and perceptive encouragement.

Dalton E. McFarland

CONTENTS

LIST OF TABLES

LIST OF FIGURES

1

MANAGERIAL INNOVATION AND

CHANGE IN THE METROPOLITAN HOSPITAL:

A CONCEPTUAL MODEL

Health care services today are provided by a complex system
of individual practitioners, health care organizations, private companies, and governments at the local, state, and federal levels. It
is more and more the case that providers work in and through
organizations, rather than as solo practitioners, to provide health
care and medical services for the ultimate consumer. Although
traditional practitioner-patient relationships remain important, the
fact that practitioners must rely heavily upon organizations for
conducting their practices has not been adequately researched.

Even solo practitioners need laboratories, pharmacies,
clinics, and hospitals for tests, drugs, and patient care. They are
often paid by insurance companies. They are guided, helped, or
inhibited by government units at local, state, and national levels.
Practitioners form professional associations which provide peer
support and review, ethical codes, spokesmanship for the group,
lobbying efforts, intercommunication, and educational services.
However, professionals and technicians work primarily in service
organizations such as partnerships, corporations, hospitals, clinics,
and the like. As early as 1958, Everett Hughes described the decline of the professional as a lone agent and his emergence as an
organization member.[1]

The proliferation of organizations within which professionals
work introduces problems of management and administration that
were nonexistent or less relevant in earlier times. No doubt, this
organizational complexity is in response to greater patient needs
and to emerging social, political, and economic policies that abhor
failures of the system to deliver adequate health care services to
all who need them. It arises also from the burgeoning technologies
of medicine and health care. It is clear that the time has come to

achieve a better understanding of the limitations and capabilities of health service organizations and to develop a better knowledge of how they are managed.

It is not sufficient to study the hospital alone. The work which resulted in this book is part of a larger design intended ultimately to analyze the health services field as a primary social institution interacting with business, government, and education. The systems nature of social institutions has a practical bearing upon organizations and the professions within them. The proliferation of health care organizations has been accompanied by the institutionalization of social, economic, and technical values, norms, practices, and policies. Yet the significant attributes of social institutions which shape health care services have been largely unexamined.

The hospital is but one subsystem in a complex health care system whose technologies, practices, norms, values, and beliefs are institutionalized in the web of society itself. The hospital cannot stand alone; it must coalesce with other subsystems of the total health care enterprise, just as the total system itself must coalesce with other social institutions.[2]

Deficiencies in the analysis of hospital problems may arise from failure to study the hospital as part of a larger sociotechnical system. Internal organizational relationships exist in a web of relationships with the external environment. For example, to explain why hospital costs are skyrocketing, we cannot fix the blame on hospitals alone. It would be a gross oversimplification to observe only internal operating efficiencies, management practices, accounting policies, and the like, for these are in part determined and affected by institutionalized forces in the surrounding sociotechnical system. We must consider laws, educational efforts, economic and political influences, the customs, values, and norms of the society, and the state of knowledge in sciences, medicine, technology, and even the arts.

The research reported in this book was conceptualized within the framework of interacting social institutions. It is an exploratory effort to examine managerial innovation and change in one type of health care organization—the general primary care metropolitan hospital. The hospital was selected as the initial focus because of the central place it occupies in the matrix of organizations and occupations which provide health care services. In the hospital, physicians, nurses, technicians, administrators, staff personnel, and patients are interacting in complex ways. The impact of the community and of public policies, as well as the convergence of economic and humanitarian forces, must all be considered; for they produce pressures, strains, and tensions which confound the emotions and affect administrators, health care workers, and patients alike.

THE SIGNIFICANCE OF INNOVATION AND CHANGE

Despite the abundant interest in innovation and change in our society, health care organizations are only just beginning to experience the need for managing more effectively for innovative, responsive change. At present, there is no single, unified, widely accepted, validated theory explaining how innovations are generated and implemented, either in organizations generally or in hospitals. We have only partial theories and tentative approaches based on a wide variety of studies, case reports, administrative investigations, and the like. Though incomplete, this mounting body of knowledge, reflected in the bibliography for this book, reveals important insights and concepts useful in developing an integrated analysis of the problems of the metropolitan hospital.

Humanity is perennially intrigued by the impact of the processes of innovation and change. Innovation intrigues us because it reflects the possibilities for continuous creativity in relation to outcomes essential to a higher quality of life, if not to humanity's survival. Innovation as practical creativity lies deep within the human psyche. It seeks constantly to be expressed, to be tested, to be appreciated. Resistance to the impulses of change is indeed often present, but it is also frequently overcome by the power of timely ideas guided by the astute administrator acting as a leader.

Innovation implies optimism and hope for the future. Even though tied to the demands of the present, people acknowledge their history and speculate about their future. This propensity for time-binding (Korzybski's phrase[3]) yields continuities that give meaning to change. The consciousness of time carries with it the implication that the future is built upon the past, but that it will be different, and that administrators and professionals may influence things for the better. If consciously innovative rather than purely accidental or adaptive changes are to occur in hospitals, they will be orchestrated by individuals who find their creative impulses nourished and utilized by their organizational milieu.

CONCEPTS AND DEFINITIONS

Technological innovation and change were excluded as a direct focus of this study. Instead, the investigations centered on administrative problems of innovation and change, many of which result from technological advances. Hospitals are high-technology organizations; thus, medical and health care technology could not be completely ignored. Yet from the perspective of managerial and organizational change, technology is instrumental. That is, it influences the nature of innovations and changes in the establishment, maintenance, and operation of the modern hospital. ✓

Mohr provides the best conceptual definition for studying innovation in the hospital: the successful introduction into an applied situation of means or ends that are new to that situation.[4] This definition, though narrower than some, was chosen to guide the field work reported on in this study. Broader definitions frequently include the concepts of inventiveness, creativity, adoption, or adaptiveness. One benefit of Mohr's definition is that it permits a distinction between the idea of innovation and the idea of invention, which is bringing something wholly new into use. Another value is its appropriateness for studying innovation in the context of an organization through the management of ends and means. A third advantage is that it points to the study of innovation as an organizational process. Fourth, it implies a process by which an organization learns what it needs to know and maintains a balance between change and stability.

Zaltman, Duncan, and Holbek define innovation as "any idea, practice, or material artifact perceived to be new by the relevant unit of adoption."[5] Similarly, but more narrowly, Rogers and Shoemaker define it as "an idea, practice, or object perceived as new by the individual."[6] The Mohr and the Zaltman, Duncan, and Holbek definitions are useful because they can be applied not only to the individual but to an organization or other grouping such as a city, community, state, or even a society or a nation. Also, they include the important concept of perception. Some members of an organization may not recognize a change as an innovation. Individual perceptions as to the innovativeness of a change, and hence their reactions to it, may vary. In this study, therefore, observations and analyses were extended to include, as do Zaltman, Duncan, and Holbek, what various individuals and adoption units perceive as innovation and change.

Change and innovation are linked together. All innovation is change, although not all change is innovation. Both affect the destinies of individuals, organizations, and social institutions. Innovation represents a creative change response to current problems and to appraisals of the emerging future. It represents adaptiveness to the demands of the environment. A hospital is innovative to the extent that its management style and structural character are open to creative change. Its organizational design, operating procedures, policies, objectives, decision processes, and managerial style and philosophy affect the generation and uses of innovation and change.

The continued existence of a hospital is reasonably assured, however, if its policies and operating procedures are sound and can accommodate routine changes. The existing structure and managerial staff can accommodate to routine change through habitual performance of planning, organizing, controlling, and other administrative functions. However, innovation beyond ordinary change is needed to cope with complex outreach and growth objectives and with the increasing turbulence and complexity of the hospital's environment.

Dynamic change is manifested in consequences that are more far-reaching and that involve wider interrelationships and more externalities than routine change. For example, when a hospital adopts a new patient visiting policy, the aftereffects are low-key and likely to have only minor impacts on the medical staff, service personnel administrators, or the organization structure. But if the hospital switches from manual record keeping to a computerized system, work and jobs throughout the organization undergo extensive change. This kind of innovation implies dynamic rather than routine change, ordinary problem-solving and caretaker management. The pace of dynamic change is also faster. It calls for leadership which continuously defines and redefines the hospital's character, purpose, and activities so as to shape a better future.[7]

INNOVATION RESEARCH

The literature on innovation in general is voluminous, although much of it deals with technological or scientific advances. This literature was examined in the early stages of the study to develop a basis for the field work. Only the most useful sources will be cited here.

Zaltman, Duncan, and Holbek provide one of the most comprehensive models of general innovative change in organizations. It focuses on the origins of change, the search processes needed to uncover alternatives, persuasion, decision and adoption processes, and implementation procedures. They test various theories and the works of other researchers against this model, concluding that there is substantial variation among researchers as to their emphasis on different parts of the model.[8]

Many studies have been devoted primarily to diffusion and adoption processes. Rothman summarizes the available research and presents several basic generalizations, together with action guidelines for practitioners. Rothman's material incorporates broad social perspectives as well as organizational factors.[9] Rogers and Shoemaker provide 193 basic generalizations about the diffusion of innovations synthesized from over 1,500 publications.[10] Havelock's extensive bibliography[11] and his report on the utilization and dissemination of knowledge[12] are extremely important. Finally, a number of landmark scholarly articles on general innovation processes are presented in a reader by <u>Rowe and Boise</u>.[13]

INNOVATION STUDIES IN HEALTH CARE ORGANIZATIONS

As was found in the case of general innovation research, diffusion and adoption were the most widely studied processes in research on innovation in health care organizations. Several of these provided useful background for this study.

In one of the most comprehensive source books on health services research, Flook and Sanazaro provide over 1,200 references and an extensive bibliography of bibliographies. This book presents sources, but only brief comments on findings. However, the sources are organized for a retrospective look at the historical development of health services research in the twentieth century through 1974, and in addition, for an examination of future prospects in this field. These citations include many works on change and innovation in health services fields, as well as on research methods, research organizations, and sources of support.[14]

Somer's study of doctors, patients, hospitals, and professional roles in the health care fields provides useful insights.[15] White's report of a conference on interorganizational research in health services emphasized interorganizational, interagency, and coordination problems.[16] The impact of social change and interpersonal relations on the diffusion of medical innovations is analyzed by Coleman et al. This study, though it focuses specifically on the diffusion of a new drug, contains valuable insights concerning the interconnections between patients and doctors, doctors and doctors, and on the process of diffusion of innovations.[17]

INNOVATION STUDIES IN HOSPITALS

Research on innovation and change in hospital contexts has been increasing, but the studies are often limited to one particular segment, such as nursing, drugs, medical care, or patient services. Many of the studies take place in psychiatric rather than general care hospitals. Georgopoulos provides an extensive review of these studies up to 1975.[18]

Two studies made in psychiatric hospitals are among the few that relate innovation and change to the organization-wide setting. The first was an extensive longitudinal study using the methods of participant observation. Greenblatt, with the aid of a social scientist and a communications specialist, observed organizational innovation and change in a large state mental hospital in 1963-67, during which time he was the hospital's superintendent. This book is rich in insights and implications for the theory of innovation and change in hospitals. One important finding was that innovation in the hospital flourishes when it is able to support an internal behavioral research organization of its own.[19]

A second valuable study is Schulman's analysis of innovation in a psychiatric hospital. He found and analyzed 131 innovations which occurred between 1954 and 1963. A longitudinal study, it also used methods of participant observation supplemented by extensive interviews, document studies, and an attitude questionnaire. This book is an excellent model for qualitative studies that generate useful insights and hypotheses.[20]

Kaluzny has provided an excellent critical review of innovation in health services organizations. His analysis of research and theory on innovation in the health care context reviews existing studies on social organization, diffusion, and adoption.[21]

Kaluzny and associates have provided a penetrating comparative study of innovation in hospitals and health departments. They investigated the differential contribution of selected organizational variables affecting the innovation of high-risk versus low-risk health service programs in the two types of organizations. They found organizational size to be a critical factor in program innovation in high-risk services in hospitals and low-risk services in health departments. Apart from size, the characteristics of the staff, such as cosmopolitan orientation and training, were prime predictors for both high- and low-risk programs in health departments and for low-risk programs in hospitals. The degree of formalization was the primary predictor of innovation in high-risk hospital programs. The cosmopolitan orientation of the administrator was a critical factor in the innovation of high-risk programs in both hospitals and health departments.[22]

Kaluzny's review of health services research concluded that five problem areas exist in innovation research: (1) commonalities among innovations, (2) communication channels, (3) factors associated with decision stages in innovation, (4) a broader conceptual framework, and (5) a longitudinal assessment of variables affecting innovation.[23] Coe has suggested the need for systems and modeling approaches to the study of innovation in hospitals. He emphasizes the need to study innovators as they carry out their work through administrative processes.[24]

The research reported in this book was designed to fill some of the gaps indicated by Kaluzny and Coe. We will now examine several current models of innovation and change, and present a conceptual model which provides for the study of innovation and change processes and the related behavior patterns of hospital administrators and other innovators.

MODELS OF INNOVATION AND CHANGE

While there is as yet no comprehensive theory of organizational innovation,[25] the basis for theoretical development exists in the form of linear process models. These models depict the principal stages by which an innovation moves from conception to testing to ultimate rejection or use. Each stage provides a focus for research and a basis for analyzing how people in organizations produce innovations. The definitions of the various stages vary, but most researchers agree that innovation occurs over time and requires a sequence of actions and decisions, each dependent on the others. There is little agreement on the number or exact nature of the postulated stages.

The earliest linear process model was presented by a committee of rural sociologists in 1955.[26] It was based on theoretical reasoning rather than on empirical research. This five-stage model of the "adoption process," depicted in Figure 1.1, became a widely held view of the innovation-decision process, serving as a guide for later empirical research.

Widely accepted at first, critics assailed the linear model as empirical research advanced. Among the chief criticisms, in addition to oversimplification, are that (1) the process does not actually end with adoption; it must allow for rejection before and after trial and for confirmation or reinforcement, and (2) the five stages are not strictly linear, as implied, in that some stages may be skipped, and some, such as evaluation, occur throughout the process rather than at a single stage. Thus the linear model is inadequate for explaining innovation processes in the hospital analyzed here, for it does not provide for key constructs, such as organization structure, problem defining, and problem solving. Also, it is based solely on the individual as an innovator rather than on organizational elements.

Rogers and Shoemaker developed the improved model shown in Figure 1.2. This model is much more complete. It incorporates both human and organizational capabilities, and includes the antecedents and consequences of an innovation. Finally, it provides for a number of alternative fates: confirmation, discontinuance, rejection, or readoption. Although any model is necessarily a simplification of reality, the Rogers and Shoemaker model is the most appropriate for studying the hospital organization, since the four

FIGURE 1.1

Traditional Linear Model of the Innovation-Decision Process

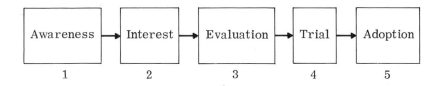

Awareness stage. The individual learns of the existence of the new idea but lacks information about it.

Interest stage. The individual develops interest in the innovation and seeks additional information about it.

Evaluation stage. The individual makes mental application of the new idea to the present and anticipated future situation and decides whether or not to try it.

Trial stage. The individual applies the new idea on a small scale or on a tentative basis in order to determine its feasibility.

Adoption stage. The individual adopts the new idea on a full scale, establishing it on a permanent basis.

Source: Adapted from North Central Rural Sociology Sub-committee for the Study of Diffusing of Farm Practices, How Farm People Accept New Ideas, Iowa Agricultural Extension Service Special Report no. 15-RS (Ames, Iowa, 1955).

9

FIGURE 1.2

Expanded Model of the Innovation-Decision Process

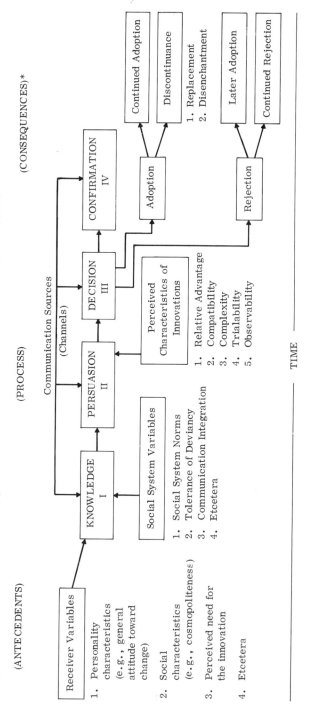

*For the sake of simplicity the diagram does not show the consequences of the innovation in this paradigm but only the consequences of the process.

Source: Everett M. Rogers and F. Floyd Shoemaker, Communication of Innovations: A Cross-Cultural Approach, 2nd ed. (New York: Free Press, 1971), p. 102. Used by permission.

10

states (knowledge, persuasion, decision, and confirmation) are applicable both to the individual and the organizational components. [27]

The matrix model shown in Figure 1.3 was constructed during the field research for this project. It reflects the processes at work in the primary research site. It adds three key elements that go beyond the Rogers-Shoemaker model: a feedback cycle, expectations, and the use of training and development in the evaluation and testing stages. The feedback cycle calls attention to the impacts of various events on one or several of the preceding stages. The concept of expectations implies an attitude or mind-set toward innovation and change that arise out of the hospital's total philosophy. The inclusion of training and development allows for the acquisition of new skills, the changing of attitudes, and the means by which an organization copes with resistance to change. This model tempers the strict sequentiality implied by earlier models. A proactive strategy for innovation and change would require particular attention to all elements and stages of this model.

CONCEPTUAL AND THEORETICAL ISSUES

There has been great instability in the empirical research findings on innovation. That is, the findings exhibit extreme variance from one study to another which prevents the results from being cumulative and inhibits the building of a general theory of organizational innovation. Progress toward what Rogers and Shoemaker call integrative theory has been slow. [28]

Downs and Mohr [29] advance four factors that explain this instability: (1) different types of innovations may have different explanations, (2) researchers have not clearly distinguished between primary and secondary attributes of innovations and/or organizations, (3) the tendency to study either single or multiple innovations per se and to ignore the relationships between innovations and the organizational setting, and (4) clouding the measurement of the dependent variable by failing to recognize that different operationalizations tap different aspects of innovation.

From their analysis of the sources of the instability of innovation research, Downs and Mohr derive seven caveats to guide research on innovation as a general phenomenon. The caveats are based on the need for measurement, the study of particular innovations, and a better typology of innovations. The caveats are summarized as follows:

1. Study different innovations to find the impact of their primary attributes (inherent characteristics) on models of innovation.

FIGURE 1.3

Feedback Model of the Innovation and Change Process

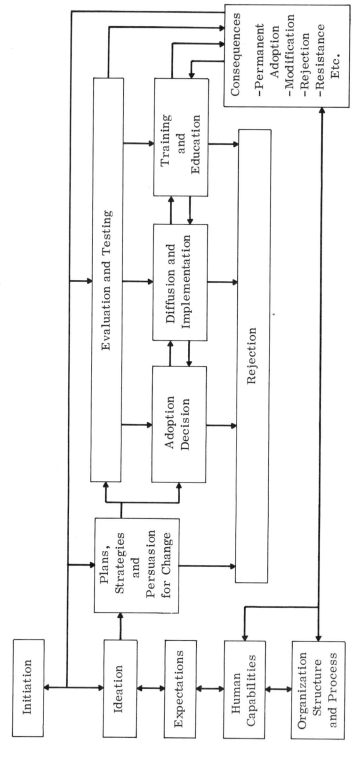

Source: Constructed by the author.

12

Observe and report the primary attributes, restricting generalizations from a given study to innovations in the same category rather than expecting all results to be identical for all
innovations.

2. Measure the secondary attributes (those perceived by the senses
   and which may be viewed differently by different perceivers).
3. Use interactive models to develop integrated theory.
4. Use the innovation-design decision (single innovation) as the
   basis for analysis, recognizing that organizational characteristics are secondary attributes (validly measured only in relation
   to a particular innovation).
5. Do not conduct multiple-innovation studies in which the organization is assigned an aggregate score for innovation.
6. Recognize that the extent of adoption and the time of adoption
   are separate concepts. Do not generalize from one variable to
   the other. Do not use either as a comprehensive measure of
   innovativeness. There is no single, unitary theory, but rather
   different theories to explain different aspects of innovation.
7. Study the adoptability of innovations by using either many innovations in a single organization or by using the innovation-
   decision design.

The research here reported followed a strategy that generally
accords with the above caveats except that, being an exploratory
study of a limited type of innovation (managerial) narrowly defined
(as a change new to the organization), it was intended to develop
propositions rather than to test them or to measure specific variables. The third caveat is met by the use of the model in Figure 1.3.
Caveats 6 and 7 are recognized in Chapter 9. The remaining caveats,
to the extent that they apply, are taken into account throughout the
book.

Pierce and Delbecq analyze innovation research in the organizational context.[30] They define innovation, following Thompson,[31] as this study does, as the generation, acceptance, and implementation of new processes, products, or services for the first
time in an organization. They argue for a conjunctive model (considering several simultaneous, interactive dimensions) rather than
a disjunctive model (where only one of a number of stimuli have to
be present). They also suggest using additive linear models rather
than a multiplicative model. The strategy of this study accords
broadly with these views, using the model in Figure 1.3, which is
both conjunctive and linear, but not additive. Pierce and Delbecq
suggest three models, one for initiation, one for adoption, and one
for implementation, on the ground that existing literature does not
provide a foundation for establishing a single predictive model. The

model shown in Figure 1.3 is a single, descriptive model which, though not predictive, yields a more comprehensive process view of innovative behavior within the organization than the Pierce and Delbecq models. Pierce and Delbecq also present 13 propositions relative to the variables in the models. These propositions will be examined, when relevant, in subsequent chapters.

METHODOLOGY OF THE STUDY

A detailed description of the research methods and problems of this study is presented in Appendix A, but a brief summary will be helpful here.

The selection of innovation and change as a focus for the field work in hospital organizations provided a rationale for viewing an array of managerial and organizational processes within the hospital. It narrowed the inquiries down to a feasible range of problems and provided an acceptable reason for the presence of researchers in the chosen sites.

The following criteria governed the selection of Victory as the primary site: (1) large size, (2) its reputation as a well-managed, successful institution, (3) the willingness of administrators to participate, and (4) a minimum of teaching, research, and religious influences.

The primary site met these criteria to differing degrees. It met the size requirement and it provided a wide array of services. Victory Hospital had a region-wide reputation for high-quality services and for excellent management. The level of interest, support, and cooperation initially and during the investigations was unusually high. In fact, the hospital had a long history of administrative studies by inside and outside researchers.

The fourth criterion was less well satisfied than the others. Victory is affiliated with a Protestant church denomination. However, denominational or religious influences appeared minimal in relation to the research objectives. Several top administrators had other denominational affiliations. Victory Hospital is not primarily a teaching institution, although it operates a school of nursing and cooperates fully with medical schools for internships and residencies. There were also training programs in medical technology, clinical and pastoral counseling, management internships, and other areas. On balance, however, the hospital met this criterion adequately for the project's needs.

Intensive field work in the primary research site was conducted from October 1, 1973 to September 30, 1975. In preparation for the main study, 8 preliminary interviews were obtained from administrators and physicians outside the focal hospital. At the main site, 17 interviews were obtained from the chief administrator and the four vice presidents; 33 department heads and supervisors and 4 staff physicians were each interviewed once, for a total of 55 interviews in Victory Hospital.

In a brief follow-up study, from late 1975 to early 1977, ten additional interviews were conducted. Two of these were with the new chief administrator at the main site, and eight were with the chief administrators of other hospitals in the same metropolitan area. This part of the study dealt primarily with boundary-spanning roles and activities by which hospitals interact with one another and with their environment. Also, the role of the regional hospital association was examined in this context.

To enter the primary and supplementary research sites armed with salient and provocative questions, the researchers examined pertinent literature on innovation in the health care system generally and on hospitals in particular. These sources are cited in the bibliography and, where appropriate, in footnotes. A preliminary set of broad, fundamental questions about innovation and change in health care organizations generally was developed. From this list, 16 question categories were derived. These questions, presented in Appendix B, relate specifically to innovation and change in hospitals.

Both the general and specific questions were used in training the two research assistants for their interviewing and analytical work and to guide the principal researcher in interviewing, analysis, observation, and the organization of research materials. An interviewing protocol was devised to (1) systematize the conduct of the interviewing, (2) guide the interviewers during the interview process, and (3) assure that key questions were introduced into all the interviews. The interview protocol is presented in Appendix C.

Depth interviewing through open-ended questions and free responses was the principal method of data collection. The interview data were supplemented by the researchers' observations in the primary field site and by the study of the hospital's records and documents. A systematic coding method was devised to analyze the resulting large volume of relatively unstructured, qualitative data. Only the interview data were coded and indexed. For this purpose, eight major categories, with their relevant dimensions, were established. These are presented in Appendix D.

In the collection of data and analyses of the findings, the researchers followed the methods suggested by Glaser and Strauss. Their concept of the constant comparative method of analysis was highly appropriate, since it provides for the continuous adjustment of data collection and analyses to the changing conditions of a dynamic, ongoing investigation. Theory building, analysis, and data collection mutually interact as the research proceeds.[32]

In presenting the interview data, informants are quoted as nearly verbatim as possible. Although recorders were not used during the interviews, the researchers recorded the informants' comments as exactly as possible immediately after each interview. The informant responses included in this book have been edited slightly to delete meaningless repetition associated with verbal discourse and to change or delete names to preserve the anonymity of people and the research site. Thus the problems of innovation and change in the hospital are expressed in the unique and realistic words of the principal actors themselves.

The two following chapters describe Victory Hospital and its organization in the context of innovation and change. Chapters 4 through 11 present a description and analysis of the major findings with respect to the matrix model presented in Figure 1.3. The final chapter reviews the implications of the study for the improvement of hospital management and presents a discussion of future directions for research on innovation and change in the management of hospitals.

NOTES

1. Everett Hughes, Men and Their Work (New York: Free Press, 1958).
2. Illich has attacked the institutionalization of health care services, professional medicine, and science in medicine in an astounding book that ignores innovations, change, and administrative processes except to decry them. He proposes an unrealistic and unworkable return to self-care by the afflicted and ill, and the withdrawal of the powers of physicians to define what constitutes illness and disease and the remedies therefor. See Ivan Illich, Medical Nemesis (New York: Random House, 1976).
3. Alfred Korzybski, Manhood of Humanity: The Art and Science of Human Engineering (New York: Dutton, 1921).
4. Lawrence B. Mohr, "Determinants of Innovation in Organizations," American Political Science Review 63 (March 1969): 111.
5. Gerald Zaltman, Robert Duncan, and Jonny Holbek, Innovations and Organizations (New York: Wiley, 1973), p. 10.
6. Everett M. Rogers and F. Floyd Shoemaker, Communication of Innovation: A Crosscultural Approach, rev. ed. of Diffusion of Innovations (New York: Free Press, 1971), p. 19.

7. The concept of innovation as dynamic change is developed in Maneck S. Wadia, "The Administrative Function of Innovation," International Review of Administrative Science 27, no. 1 (1961): 324-28.

8. Zaltman, Duncan, and Holbek, op. cit.

9. Jack Rothman, Planning and Organizing for Social Change (New York: Columbia University Press, 1974), Ch. 9.

10. Rogers and Shoemaker, op. cit.

11. Ronald G. Havelock, Bibliography on Knowledge Utilization and Dissemination (Ann Arbor: Center for Research on Utilization of Scientific Knowledge, Institute for Social Research, University of Michigan, 1968).

12. Ronald G. Havelock, Planning for Utilization Through Dissemination and Utilization of Knowledge (Ann Arbor: Institute for Social Research, University of Michigan, 1969).

13. Lloyd Rowe and William B. Boise, eds., Organizational and Managerial Innovation (Pacific Palisades, Calif.: Goodyear Publishing Company, 1973).

14. E. Evelyn Flook and Paul J. Sanazaro, Health Services Research and R D in Perspective (Ann Arbor, Mich.: Health Administration Press, 1973).

15. Ann R. Somer, Health Care in Transition: New Directions for the Future (Chicago: Hospital Research and Educational Trusts, 1971).

16. Paul W. White, ed., Interorganizational Research on Health (Springfield, Va.: National Technical Information Service, 1971).

17. James S. Coleman, Elihu Katz, and Herbert Menzel, Medical Innovation: A Diffusion Study (Indianapolis, Ind.: Bobbs-Merrill, 1966).

18. Basil S. Georgopoulos, Hospital Organization Research: Review and Source Book (Philadelphia: W. B. Saunders, 1975).

19. Milton Greenblatt, Myron R. Sharaf, and Evelyn M. Stone, Dynamics of Institutional Change (Pittsburgh: University of Pittsburgh Press, 1971).

20. J. Schulman, Remaking an Organization: Innovation in a Specialized Psychiatric Hospital (Albany: State University of New York Press, 1969).

21. Arnold D. Kaluzny, "Innovation of Health Services: Theoretical Framework and Review of Research," Health Services Research, Summer 1974, pp. 101-20.

22. Arnold D. Kaluzny, James E. Veney, and John T. Gentry, "Innovation of Health Services: A Comparative Study of Hospitals and Health Departments," Health and Society 52 (Winter 1974): 51-82.

23. Kaluzny, op. cit., pp. 101-20.

24. Rodney M. Coe, ed., Planned Change in the Hospital: Case Studies of Organizational Innovations (New York: Praeger, 1970), Chs. 1 and 8.

25. Harvey M. Sapolsky, "Organizational Structure and Innovation," Journal of Business 40, no. 4 (October 1967): 497-510.

26. North Central Rural Sociology Subcommittee for the Study of Diffusing of Farm Practices, How Farm People Accept New Ideas, Iowa Agricultural Extension Service Special Report no. 15-RS (Ames, Iowa, 1955).

27. Rogers and Shoemaker, op. cit., pp. 101-04.

28. Ibid., p. 346.

29. George W. Downs, Jr., and Lawrence B. Mohr, "Conceptual Issues in the Study of Innovation," Administrative Science Quarterly 21 (December 1976): 700-14.

30. Jon L. Pierce and André L. Delbecq, "Organization Structure, Individual Attitudes, and Innovation," Academy of Management Review 2 (January 1977): 27-37.

31. Victor A. Thompson, "Bureaucracy and Innovation," Administrative Science Quarterly 10 (January 1965): 1-20.

32. Barney Glaser and Anselm Strauss, The Discovery of Grounded Theory (Chicago: Aldine, 1967).

2

VICTORY HOSPITAL:

STRUCTURE, LEADERSHIP, AND

SUCCESSION OF OFFICE

Our analysis of managerial innovation and change necessarily begins with a review of the organizational context in which the field observations were made. We will first describe the structural characteristics of Victory Hospital, the main site of this study. We will then examine two challenges the Victory organization faced in order to illustrate the dynamic forces at work which had substantial impacts on change and innovation.

THE NORFIELD MEDICAL COMPLEX

To understand the organization of Victory Hospital it is necessary to examine the larger framework of which it is a part. Victory is one of two major hospitals in a multi-unit organization known as the Norfield Medical Complex. The parent organization consists of a central group of administrative officers and staff service personnel and a board of trustees. It operates, in addition to Victory, a 450-bed general care, short-stay institution known as Bright Hospital.

Both hospitals are similar in size but located several miles apart in the same metropolitan area. They are both voluntary, short-stay, primary care institutions in the private, not-for-profit sector. While Bright and Victory are the main units, Norfield also has contractual management service agreements with two other smaller hospitals. Norfield has been active in joint projects with a number of health-related organizations, including the provision of land and other facilities required by their collaborations. Development activities have been extensive in Norfield since the organization's inception in 1922 as a single 90-bed hospital. Older buildings were acquired, renovated, and new ones built. In 1973, the central offices were relocated to a newly acquired building located approximately midway between Victory and Bright hospitals.

The Norfield organization is infused with a spirit of entrepreneurial planning for growth based on concepts of community involvement and service. At the time of this study it had become the largest hospital complex anywhere in the world under the ownership of a local religious denomination, and the ninth largest not-for-profit hospital complex in the nation in the number of patients served. It is the largest hospital complex in its state, and it continues to grow, as reflected in its extensive physical facilities, land holdings, and development plans. On the Victory Hospital premises are a 500-bed hospital building, a classroom and housing facility for 200 students in the School of Nursing, a 425-car parking deck, a seven-story professional office building, and other structures resulting from its collaboration with other groups. All these are located on a 142-acre wooded tract with ample space for expansion. Some of the land is devoted to an office park development. The premises throughout are attractively landscaped. Bright Hospital has a building with 450 beds, a professional office building, a 400-car parking lot, and an award-winning garden park.

In 1975, Norfield's assets totaled nearly $70 million. Its operating budget approached $44 million. An affiliated denominational foundation had assets of more than $600,000, and it aggressively raises funds to support Norfield's widespread activities. Norfield had 2,800 employees, nearly 36,000 bed patients, and over 500 physicians on its medical staffs. It also had over 750,000 visitors, 2,300 babies born, 40,000 emergency patients, and 450 volunteer workers. It conducted nearly 400,000 laboratory tests, over 38,000 x-ray procedures, 17,000 surgical operations, 125,000 heart procedures, and 98,000 physical therapy treatments. The average patient stay in Norfield's two hospitals is eight and one-half days.

Norfield's entrepreneurial thrust is evident in its plans for the future, which include the construction of retirement apartments for the elderly, custodial care units for those unable to care for themselves, and within a decade, a third "campus" of 40 acres in an adjacent county, to consist of a 300-bed hospital, a professional office building, extended care facilities, and a nursing home. Its proactive strategies have resulted in management assistance contracts with two smaller nearby hospitals, innovative affiliations with nearby public and private universities, and collaboration with private associations. Norfield and its affiliates already cover three counties, and it contemplates expansion into other counties as well, through mergers, purchases, management contracts, affiliation agreements, or new construction. According to Robert Manton, the president at the time this study began:

We firmly believe—and a lot of people don't agree with us—that the little hospitals can't offer everything the public needs anymore. . . . At the Norfield Medical Complex, we're trying to put together a group of hospitals under one management that can share the experts and services we have. . . . No longer can we think just in terms of single hospitals. . . . For one thing, small hospitals can't afford the top-quality people that larger groups of hospitals can hire. And you can't run a first-class institution with second-class people. . . . We can afford the people we need, if we can share them.

An example of Norfield's propensity for affiliation is the merger in 1973 of its nursing school with the school of nursing at a nearby university. A further example, with a private association, occurred in 1974 when Norfield successfully won a bid to provide the location (on the Victory premises) of a new private national speech and hearing center. Finally, the entrepreneurial attitude is reflected in a U. S. Department of Health, Education, and Welfare Grant in 1975 to make a six-month, two-county study of the need for a Health Maintenance Organization, and a review of the extent to which family doctors and medical clinics are meeting the health care needs of people in the two counties.

The headquarters staff consists of 50 officers, administrators, clerical, and computer personnel. The president heads a central office team consisting of vice presidents of finance, community relations, and facilities planning, an executive engineer, and the two chief administrators in charge of Bright and Victory, and a number of program directors specializing in health care technologies. A board of trustees is the principal governing body of the central Norfield organization and its hospitals and other units.

The rationale of the multi-unit structure at Norfield is to provide efficient planning, direction, and control and centralized services such as computer work, personnel activities, purchasing, and finance. The central staff also devotes substantial resources to policy matters, community relations, capital budgeting, long-range planning and development, and major problems such as labor relations.

The Norfield organization resembles the "multihospital holding company," described by Platou and Rice as analogous to bank holding companies. They depict the multi-unit structure as an organizational innovation that achieves economies of scale and improvements in data processing, materials management, budgetary forecasting, systematic decision making, operations research, and

long-range planning.[1] Although the studies at Victory generally
support this rationale, it was also found that there are difficulties
of coordination and communication in multi-unit operations that
should not be minimized. Managers at all levels in Victory reported conflicts in their relationships with the central group. It
appears, therefore, that the optimism of Platou and Rice must be
tempered by the fact that multi-unit structures are not a simple
solution to the problems of hospital care on rising costs.

Nevertheless, the Norfield organization provides Victory Hospital with leadership, services, policy guidance, goals, and plans—
resources it would not otherwise have. The resulting adventurous
spirit is demanding, but it has generated feelings of pride within the
Victory organization and an outstanding reputation in the community.

THE ORGANIZATION OF VICTORY HOSPITAL

Victory Hospital was established in 1952, replacing an older
hospital at another site which had been operated by the denomination since 1930. It opened the new facilities on the present site in
1966, when its present organization structure was established.

At the time of this study, the physical facilities were modern
and designed to provide a wide range of patient care services. In
addition to the 500 beds for medical-surgical patients, it had three
intensive care units covering medical, surgical, and coronary care.
It also had a maternity department and nurseries, a pediatric unit,
a diabetes and metabolic unit, a short-term psychiatric unit, and an
emergency unit. It provided support services in pathology, clinical
laboratories, radiology, physical therapy, and inhalation therapy.
Victory also had a cardiovascular diagnostic laboratory and facilities
for open-heart surgery. Victory was the first private or community
hospital in its state to perform open-heart surgery, and the first to
have a cobalt unit. It was equipped with closed-circuit radio and
television systems for educational and patient information purposes.

Occupancy rates at Victory have remained consistently above
the 90 percent level. The spirit of entrepreneurship has resulted
in successful projects that extend beyond the confines of ordinary
hospital administration. This attitude, coupled with relatively abundant organizational resources, has helped to forge innovative exten-
sions of the organization's service capabilities.

Victory's problems, however, arose from its very success.
It has a substantially larger property management problem than
most hospitals of its type, since its holdings in urban land, buildings, and facilities are extensive. Like other hospitals, it has
problems of fighting inflationary costs, maintaining effectiveness

and efficiency, and keeping up with the advancing technology of health care. During the study, federal price controls for hospitals increased the pinch of inflation, and top officials of the parent organization lobbied hard in Congress for the removal of these controls.

Victory Hospital, whatever its problems and deficiencies, exhibited an aura of success. This is reflected in the way organization members perceived challenge and opportunity in their work, by its prestige in the community, and by the positive evaluations of patients and the medical staff. Employees at all levels exhibited a strong sense of mission and feelings of pride and accomplishment. They viewed their work not only as a matter of technical effectiveness but also in terms of its human and social impacts.

The structural hierarchy is relatively flat, consisting of four main levels. The first level consists of the chief administrator and the positions in his office; the second level consists of the vice presidents and positions in their offices; the third level consists of the main department heads. Within departments, there is a fourth level of supervisory managers heading the functionally defined internal units appropriate to each of these domains.

Figure 2.1 is a chart of the Victory organization. It was headed by the chief administrator, William Wright. Reporting to him were Alice Winters, vice president of nursing; Lora Nelling, vice president for business administration; and Ben Watson and Dale Ellis, each a vice president in charge of a group of operating departments. In addition, the chaplain reported directly to Wright. This top management group was the focus of a major portion of the interviews.

Structurally, Victory Hospital exhibited no major departures from hospital organization typical for its size. There were parallel structures for the administrative and the medical staffs. Within Victory, the nursing group was the largest unit, consisting of over 600 persons in the various categories of nursing service. There were no major structural innovations in evidence, but substantial flexibility of attitudes toward organization design prevailed among the top managers.

We are now ready to consider the two major sets of events which challenged the Victory organization. The first consisted of a severe episode of labor strife, and the second was a series of traumatic resignations by top administrators in Norfield and in Victory. Both challenges revealed Victory's ability to cope with adversity, and both reflect the dynamics of change with respect to the organization itself.

FIGURE 2.1

Organization Structure of Victory Hospital

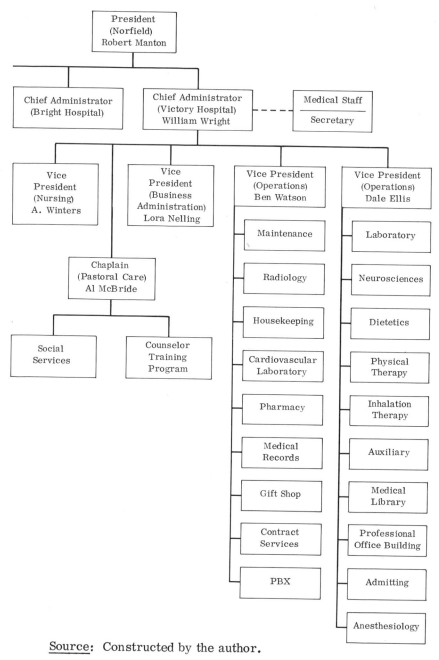

Source: Constructed by the author.

LABOR STRIFE

Shortly after the study began, both Bright and Victory hospitals were the target of a union organization drive focused on their kitchen and maintenance personnel and licensed practical nurses. The main thrust was at Bright, but the struggle spilled over into Victory's domain. The administrators at Norfield, Bright, and Victory regarded the move as an invasion by external forces, and hence took steps to fend off the attacks.

The task of coping fell primarily to the administrators of Bright and Victory, since there were no labor specialists in either hospital or in the central office. Advice as well as help was available only through "outsiders" remote from firing-line problems, instead of from specialists in labor relations integrated into the management structure. Thus, it was unclear from the start whether the same approaches to labor problems should be followed at both Bright and Victory, or whether each should go its own way, with the central office playing only a low-key advisory role. Indeed, no one could let the problems alone; everyone got into the act. Trustees and the central office staff were concerned with personnel matters and provided advice, but the net effect was to place the pressure on the two administrators who in turn relied heavily upon the vice presidents and the heads of departments and other units. Thus, everyone had to devote full attention to the labor problem. "Night and day we had time for little else" was a frequent report. The intense preoccupation throughout the organization with labor problems was short but intense, with the result that innovation and change were curtailed.

Although the walkouts and picketing were more extensive at Bright, the managers at Victory first overreacted, reducing innovation. As the strife wore on, however, an opposite reaction emerged:

Interviewer: Are you concerned more with day-to-day
   activities than you think is good for innovation?
Nelling: Yes. There is a lot of day-to-day pressure
   here. Sometimes we overdo it. . . . When the
   picketing lasted, we realized we had gone too far,
   so we pulled away.
Interviewer: In what way?
Nelling: We just quit spending so much energy on
   watching the picketers and nursing our fears about
   all manner of consequences. We had everyone here
   working night and day for weeks. This we realized
   was a bad allocation of time, so we backed away
   from it.

Another reaction to the labor problems that was harmful to innovation at Victory was the centralization of certain personnel functions formerly allocated to department heads: grievance handling and the discharge of employees were taken from department heads and moved to the vice presidents' and the administrator's levels. For example, the manager of food services, in which a large number of the striking employees had worked, reported that:

> Well, needless to say, the strike has caused problems. We can't fire anybody any more in this department without going through grievance procedure. The higher-ups handle all these problems now. I believe we had seven people that quit during the strike and they were temporarily replaced for a short time. I believe the wording in the letter that administration sent these people was that "your position has been temporarily filled." It was a real touchy situation for a while, but I believe later these individuals were actually fired. When tensions were high, certain problems were brought on by the fact that people were scared and were being bullied by the union. . . . The net result of all the union problems . . . has been a shift in authority in that we can no longer fire a person although we can still hire them.

Victory was ill-equipped to deal with this threat by itself. Indeed, it did not have to do so since Norfield carried the burden of defense for both Victory and Bright. However, the Norfield organization too was inexperienced in combating unionism, with a resulting heavy reliance upon attorneys and consultants.

Figure 2.1 reveals that Victory had no formal department of employee or labor relations; in most organizations of similar size this function is important enough to be located close to the top administrator. Consequently, the problem of coping with the labor difficulties within Victory fell mainly on the chief administrator, the two operations vice presidents, and the vice president for business administration.

The trouble began on February 20, 1974 at 11 p.m. with a strike of over 140 kitchen and maintenance people and licensed practical nurses at Bright. The workers were striking for recognition of the union, but administrators refused to discuss the matter, since at that time hospitals were not included under the Taft-Hartley Act. By August 25, however, federal legislation extended the act to include hospitals, so that the dispute then came under the aegis of the National Labor Relations Board. However, the union drive was unsuccessful and ultimately lost its momentum, though not without several instances of violence.

The striking workers at Bright had been discharged for not reporting to work. Picket lines were established at both hospitals. About 20 of Victory's 1,300 nonmanagerial employees also went on strike and were similarly discharged. The violence reported in the press included the burning of homes and automobiles, shotgun blasts through windows, tire slashing, and threats of bodily injury to those crossing picket lines. Several former employees of Bright and a union official were arrested after a running gun battle and charged with attempted arson and murder.

For Victory, the consequences of the organizing drive were relatively minor and short term. Yet for over nine months they produced continuing tensions and concern within the management group. With the aid of Norfield's central group and its consultants, strategies were devised for coping both with daily events and longer-run prospects for unionization. The chief administrators at both hospitals took pride in keeping their units operating at virtually full capacity without adverse effects on patients, but the organizing drives, though unsuccessful, left a residue of anxiety which pervaded the entire system long after the immediate threats expired.

The entire management group committed enormous amounts of time and energy to their coping activities. Coping with the union drive as a perceived threat so completely occupied the time of key managers that innovation and change efforts were severely curtailed. Indeed, their main preoccupation centered on preventing a potential change originating from outside that was deemed undesirable to the organization. The union drive thus encountered a united front on the part of the managers who opposed it.

CHANGES IN LEADERSHIP

The labor-management struggle just described had limited, relatively short-term impacts on innovation and change, but a series of resignations by key administrators in both Norfield and Victory were far more serious and impinged more heavily on innovation and change.

Near the end of the projected field work, key informants departed one after another. Remaining administrators experienced changes in tasks and roles. The tenor of the hospital shifted from stability to one of temporary adjustments. These changes disrupted the cohesiveness of the two organizations, reducing innovative activity and slowing other types of change while the organizations coped with problems of staffing over a period of nearly a year. Fortunately, the researchers were permitted to extend their interviewing to incorporate the effects of these changes.

The changes formed a chain pattern not uncommon in business firms: when a key official resigns, a wave of other resignations often follows. The resignation of Robert Manton as the head of the Norfield complex triggered a wave of resignations in Norfield and in Victory Hospital although not at Bright. To understand this pattern, it is necessary first to examine the Norfield resignations, and then to describe related events in Victory.

Conventional wisdom in organizations values teamwork, cohesion, and stability amidst growth, yet at the same time recognizes that changes are unavoidable. The changes at Norfield and at Victory, however, went far beyond routine expectations of change. The existing stability provided a stark contrast to the disruptions evoked by the patterns of change that began with Manton's resignation.

The top administrative group at Norfield in 1973 and 1974 was a tightly knit, cohesive working team. These managers had worked together for nearly eight years. Members of the team were aware of each other's strengths, weaknesses, philosophies, and idiosyncracies. They had developed comfortable working styles. Three of them had worked together previously in another organization, coming to Norfield at Manton's invitation. Manton was a dynamic administrator with a national reputation in his field. He had been with Norfield for nine years, during which he was active in community affairs, a prominent spokesman for hospitals in Congress, and a leader on the state and national hospital scene. He was admired and respected by his colleagues, and his resignation produced shock waves throughout the organization.

Shortly after Manton's resignation, Norfield's board of trustees announced the appointment of Leonard Hayfield as acting president. Hayfield also continued as vice president of finance in the central office. He had been with Norfield for nine years, having been hired by Manton shortly after his arrival. Speculations naturally ensued about whether Hayfield would be appointed permanently, but after a delay of nearly eight months the board appointed a new president from outside the Norfield group. Meanwhile, this delay fostered confusion and uncertainty throughout the organization. According to Wright:

> We've had a great deal of organizational upheaval and turmoil here since Mr. Manton resigned. As you know, when a change of this kind occurs, there is a bumping effect throughout the organization and it may lead to more changes. Those changes are still under discussion and while so far you have been examining a stable organization, it is now unstable and may get more so in the future.

In the weeks following Manton's resignation and the temporary appointment of Hayfield as president, additional resignations followed both in Norfield and Victory, bearing out Wright's predictions. At Norfield, the vice president for personnel and the vice president for planning and development resigned, the former joining Manton at his new post and the latter taking a position in another state. A few weeks later Manton's former administrative assistant also left to join him on his new job. The Norfield vacancies were filled by the temporary expedients—the assignment of Hayfield to the presidency and shifting the wage and salary administrator to the duties of the departed vice president for personnel.

In Victory, there was great consternation over the changes at Norfield. Wright was clearly a possible successor to Manton; he and those on his staff were keenly aware of this. The wave of resignations that subsequently occurred was linked to the fate of Wright. Hayfield's appointment bought the board of trustees time to consider persons other than Wright, who became restless over the delay in clarifying his future. He decided to press the issue with the board by setting in early January of 1975 a three-week deadline for their decision about him.

When the deadline came without favorable action, Wright resigned, announcing that he would be joining Manton in his new post. During the next month, Vice President Ellis resigned, followed a few weeks later by the resignation of Vice President Watson. Both took jobs in other states, being disaffected by the many uncertainties in the organization. When it became apparent that no one from Victory would succeed to the presidency of Norfield, the chain of resignations in Victory began. After Wright's departure, it also became clear that no one from Victory would succeed him, and the two operating vice presidents departed.

The last change in top management at Victory occurred almost a year later, and six months after the selection of Wright's successor. Mrs. Winters, the vice president of nursing, resigned. Four out of five of the top officials at Victory had thus departed within a one-year period. An interview with one of the nurses taken shortly after Winters resigned disclosed that she had been an unpopular administrator, having done things not in accord with her verbal postures. "She talked democracy and receptivity to ideas, but in practice was a real martinet," according to the nurse, who also reported that Robert Grepman, who in the meantime had been named to Wright's position, welcomed the opportunity to replace her. Winters's replacement was the only one of the three major vacancies at Victory that was filled from the inside.

Following the resignations of Wright, Ellis, and Watson, it was uncertain whether the board would delay appointing Wright's successor until a permanent replacement for Manton was found.

Hayfield urged the board to fill the Victory position as quickly as possible; and within a few weeks it hired Robert Grepman. According to Hayfield:

> Mr. Grepman was an excellent choice for Victory. At first I was a little skeptical whether we should fill the position until Manton's successor had a chance to review everything and help make the choice. On the other hand, we had lost Ellis and Watson, and things were rather hectic around Victory right then. So I encouraged the board to fill the slot anyway. When Mr. Grepman was interested in the job, I told him that he was going to have his work cut out for him there for a while. . . . After he came, I told him that we would help him all we could but that we were short-handed over here too. . . . I recommended that he fill the two vice presidential vacancies there as soon as possible. However, he said he wanted to study everything, get acquainted with the department heads, and take the time to make careful decisions.

THE TRAUMA OF CHANGE

The changes in Norfield's central organization induced traumatic changes in Victory. Feelings of shock and surprise swept through the organization, followed by anxiety and uncertainty on the part of those still remaining. As the chain of resignations continued, the level of concern and doubt increased, and every manager had to assess the impacts of the changes on his own career.

The traumatic effects were due more to the breaking up of friendships and alliances than to the disruption of operations. At the time of these changes, the top managers and their positions at Victory were relatively new. Wright was the most senior, having been hired by Manton nine years earlier to head the Victory organization at its new location. But the two operating vice presidents, Ellis and Watson, and the vice president of business administration, Mrs. Nelling, had been in office less than two years. Winters had been with the nursing group eight years, but had been a vice president for only three. Despite this relatively young group, substantial cohesiveness had developed among its members. Consequently, the domino effect was all the more startling as the key leaders in Victory relinquished their positions. At the time of Manton's resignation, Ellis had guardedly but prophetically predicted these changes in Victory: "We are just beginning to feel cohesive [pause] maybe that means it's time for a change around here!"

The fact that Victory's services were so little affected by these traumatic changes was due to the willingness of the remaining managers to shift their duties and accept temporary reallocations of responsibility, and to the stability of the cadres of department heads and supervisory managers at lower levels. The primary impact of the resignations and shifts of responsibility was on the increased anxiety and unrest which came to pervade the organization and on the level of innovation and change which fell in the face of the maintenance patterns that evolved.

Ellis described the impact of the changes on feelings and relationships, and the resulting pressure to reassess careers, as follows:

> Ellis: Bill Wright's resignation is going to hit us
> hard, and me in particular. He was loved as an
> administrator here and I was very close to him
> personally. I can understand why he wants to
> leave. He was close to Manton, and when Manton
> resigned, it left him with an ambiguous relation-
> ship in the central office. Besides, he says he has
> accomplished all he can in his present position, and
> to make a greater contribution he would have to
> have a direct relationship with the board of trust-
> ees, and not have to go through the president. He
> didn't care so much whether he got Mr. Manton's
> job or not, but he did want to work directly with
> the doctors and hospital people on the one hand and
> the board of trustees on the other. So everything
> was in limbo for a while.
>
> Interviewer: So it has been a rather traumatic time?
>
> Ellis: Yes. In hospitals we are extremely people-
> oriented. We get used to liking each other. It's
> kind of a family love affair here and interpersonal
> relations are very important. We haven't had a
> lot of changes in people and therefore this is making
> a lot of people feel sad.
>
> Interviewer: What do you think will be some of the
> effects of Mr. Wright's departure?
>
> Ellis: Right now we are in the middle of an extensive
> organization upheaval and there is more to come.
> I think you'll see others leaving. Ben Watson and
> I both have to think about what this place will be
> like and whether we will want to continue. There
> will be changes in the general office to take into
> account. Who knows what six months will bring?

> Maybe I'll be ready to move on, or maybe I'll stay
> and have a better job here.
>
> Interviewer: You feel you have some lead time for
> planning?
>
> Ellis: Yes, I think it's good not to rush these chain
> reactions. It's very traumatic, and even if people
> move quite a bit, it is good not to have it all hap-
> pen at once. But the key changes are quite painful.
> Bill Wright was like a brother to me, a very dear
> friend, and it looks like he will be leaving not only
> Victory but the city too. It's hard to adjust to the
> shock when you're right in the middle of trying to
> figure it out.

That changes of a similar nature did not also occur in Bright
Hospital is attributable to the fact that in Victory the top administrators had closer working relationships with Manton, having worked
with him elsewhere. Also, the administrator at Bright was older,
less concerned about advancing his career outside or within Norfield, and was not a prime contender for Manton's position. With
Bright's administrator remaining at Bright, there were no change
pressures directly at work in that part of the organization.

Ellis's resignation was followed shortly after that of the other
operations vice president, Ben Watson. The effect of delays in appointing successors to Manton and Wright ultimately took their toll.
Wright himself indicated this, explaining (contrary to the statement
by Ellis) that he had hoped to be Manton's successor:

> Wright: It will be announced today that Watson is leav-
> ing to become the associate administrator of a hos-
> pital in Texas. We are getting a chain reaction after
> the departure of Mr. Manton. A lot of it comes
> from the continued uncertainty. It was known that I
> hoped to be named to Mr. Manton's job. When they
> made the acting appointment, this left people with
> doubts. I think it was a mistake for the board to
> make this temporary appointment and to delay in
> finding a good replacement for Mr. Manton. He
> left on December 1, so that's . . . almost five
> months of coasting. Naturally, other people such
> as myself began to reflect on what this meant to
> their careers. When my departure was announced,
> this caused the others to think about their careers,
> too. . . . When the organization hears about Ben's
> leaving it'll be in turmoil again, and morale will
> get worse.

THE RUMOR MILL

As the impact of the changes extended throughout the organization, the trauma was intensified by rumors pervading the organization at Victory:

> Interviewer: Was this matter of Mr. Wright's resignation on the grapevine before the decision was really made?
>
> Ellis: Oh boy, yes, it sure was. There were actually two rumors. One was, who's next? The first tendency is not to like that kind of change and to think that it is not going to be good. People worried about the bums that might be brought in to take his place and all that.
>
> Interviewer: That's understandable, isn't it?
>
> Ellis: Yes, I think so, but another kind of rumor I didn't expect at all. Even was down as far as the housekeepers, they said "What's the hidden agenda?" They want to know what's going on. They think it's a conspiracy—not against them necessarily, but they think the whole thing has been rigged for some purpose that will affect them. They think it's calculated. What's going on I think is fear of the unknown. These people would rather have something bad that they know, or even have me or Ben Watson get Manton's job, more than they would a person from the outside. The unknown is the worst thing for them.
>
> Interviewer: The rumors were numerous and essentially accurate?
>
> Ellis: I think that's O.K. for management. There were a lot of rumors the regular employees didn't hear, and they didn't believe the rumors they did hear. The change was so great that they couldn't believe what they were hearing. The feelings run really deep and whether matters are factual or not, feelings are the important thing.

Wright, also, was aware of the impact of the rumor mill:

> Interviewer: Did the rumor mill function before you actually made your decision?
>
> Wright: Yes, I think it did. Naturally, people are going to speculate and talk about what they think is happening. They can put two and two together and

see what the possibilities are. I'm sure they were
not terribly surprised when I decided to leave.
Now they are going through another time of uncertainty.

Nelling also commented on the rumors, implying that she too
had been included as a subject:

Nelling: The rumors were really flying around the organization. As soon as Mr. Manton announced his
resignation, people began to speculate about who
else would be going. The rumor mill predictions
were accurate for the three people who left Victory, plus one more that we had in the rumor mill
about which nothing has happened yet.

PROBLEMS OF SUCCESSION

The loss of almost the entire top management team at both
Norfield and Victory, with replacements spread over a nine-month
period, had detrimental effects on innovation and change. These
effects were intensified by the fact that the ultimate appointees were
so different in temperament, outlook, and administrative styles.
Manton and Wright had similar administrative styles which were
aggressive, expansionist, dynamic, and proactive. They both believed in team building, and they tended to build cohesive teams of
persons similar to themselves and to form close personal relationships with them.

The explanation of why none of the team members succeeded
to the top positions in Norfield and Victory is to be found in two sets
of factors: (1) internal politics and (2) a shift of direction and
emphasis on the part of the board of trustees.

Ellis was the logical internal successor to Wright, but his
candidacy was successfully blocked by Winters, the vice president
of nursing. Two years earlier, Ellis had left a consulting firm at
a salary cut of $10,000 to join Wright. This situation added to his
impulse to consider outside opportunities. One informant in a position to know stated that if Ellis had succeeded Wright, the rest of
the chain reaction might not have occurred.

The shift in direction and emphasis of the board was evident
in the replacements ultimately hired. Research supports the theory
that control (leadership) of an organization varies depending on the
important contingencies it has to confront. One study of succession
in 57 hospitals found that size was positively related to inside

succession, to the amount of formal training in hospital administration, and to the occupational background of chief administrators. However, in accounting for the characteristics and tenure of administrators, a more important relationship was found between succession and organizational context variables. The study suggested that the effects of context are mediated through the operation of critical organizational uncertainties and contingencies. Contextual factors determine the uncertainties and problems confronted by the organization. Administrator characteristics and tenure are, in turn, related to these organizational contingencies.[2]

The wave of resignations was itself a contingency for the board. The two main hospitals had already successfully weathered the union drive. Beyond the resignations themselves, there was considerable unrest and uncertainty among department heads and their staffs. These uncertainties were increased by the board's unexplained delays in finding replacements. The ultimate result of the hiring process was again to obtain two administrators, one for Norfield and one for Victory, of the same type of management styles, but this time with a difference: instead of being aggressive and proactive, as were Manton and Wright, the two new administrators were deliberate, calm, quiet, low-profile types. A key informant sized up the new president of Norfield, Tom Ross, in the following account:

> Interviewer: Has much changed with the advent of the new head of Norfield?
> Informant: In a way it changed and in a way it didn't. Our organization structure has remained basically the same. But the management style changed a lot. The new president is much more careful and methodical than Manton. He is devoted to the idea of studying things. He uses a lot of consultants, but he uses them to verify things that we already know should be done. He is great on details, especially in the operating units.
> Interviewer: Does this tend to build confidence in the leadership?
> Informant: Not as much as you would think. You've got to remember we have a very conservative board. This top management style makes a great difference to the board. They like it. But it doesn't make much difference to the medical staff nor to the management staff as far as confidence is concerned. As administrators, we are all caught in the pressure between the board on one side and the management group on the other.

THE SLOWING OF CHANGE AND INNOVATION

Changes as traumatic and extensive as those at Norfield and Victory were widely perceived as slowing the processes of innovation and change. Asked whether the changes at Norfield affected innovation and change at Bright, the chief administrator replied:

> Yes, they did. Innovation and change depend heavily on the management style, and that changed. For example, if your management style is like mine, you're interested in people more than the institution and I think the obvious doesn't need to be studied as much as we have to study it. We waste a lot of money on consultants and research to make studies of whether something should be done instead of how it should be done.

At Victory also there were changes in management style. The new administrator and the two vice presidents he subsequently hired were conservative in their styles. They became extremely busy with day-to-day details. Clearly, the organization viewed this contingency of succession as a need to consolidate, slow down, integrate, and conduct operations efficiently. Thus, innovation and change shifted from their high priority under Wright to one of deliberate, even cautious, management under Grepman.

The changes in top leadership seriously inhibited innovation and other types of change at Victory. A holding pattern emerged in which attention was centered on filling the vacant positions and on the building of defenses by those remaining. The slowing pace of change was described by Ellis shortly before announcing his own resignation:

> Interviewer: Will these traumatic changes affect innovation or other kinds of change?
> Ellis: Certainly things will slow down. We will all turn inward a great deal. Reacting to these changes has taken up a lot of time. It took over two months to settle Bill Wright's leaving. The possibilities after Manton's resignation have set people to talking and wondering a lot. This diverts their time. It was similar to the situation we had last year when the strike was called against us. It was on our minds all the time and we took a couple of months thinking about it, reacting to it, and doing what the strike threat called for. Yet I hope we

can hold our ground in spite of this. I know that I
myself am less productive. I'm not sure what the
ground rules are going to be. Also, we can't make
any major commitments to anything right now so
we are in a state of limbo. A change like this does
create some new and different activities but not
ones that help us progress. We have to stay in a
steady state and hope to hold our own.

Interviewer: I see.

Ellis: The same thing is true for Leonard Hayfield
in the central office. He needs time to get hold of
the job, so he can't push much of anything right
at first. . . .

THE HOLDING PATTERN AS A COPING MECHANISM

The holding pattern that ensued from the wave of resignations
was a means of coping with the threatened instability of the organization. The pattern consisted of consolidating existing strengths,
and of drawing upon remaining talents for temporary realignments
of responsibilities.

In Norfield, the last of the major changes was the resignation
of Al Mann, the director of personnel. He left to join Manton and
Wright in their new posts. Fred Summer was named the acting
director of personnel. He described the resource base of the holding pattern as follows:

We have a solid organization despite the missing
people. The organization has been running quite
smoothly. That's because people have learned to
work together. Also, we still have good division
heads like Mrs. Nelling and Mrs. Winters.

Summer also paid tribute to Wright, whom he credited for paving
the way for the continuation of the Victory organization by skillful
delegating:

Summer: Delegation had a lot to do with their coping.
Mr. Wright was a great delegator and I think this
proves the wisdom of his delegation.

Interviewer: So the effects of the personnel changes
haven't been all that great?

Summer: Well, right now we are in a holding pattern.
What happens in a case like this is that you don't
do any more expanding. Your plans for growth
and development are in escrow so to speak until
the new leaders come aboard and we figure out
what we're supposed to be doing next. For example, my own work as salary administrator is
greatly reduced because we get fewer requests
from Victory. They are clearly in a holding pattern.

Ellis also observed the holding pattern, and recognized that it
would stop innovative efforts:

Yes, a lot of people are in a real tailspin right now.
But our general administration will be O.K. We'll
all continue doing about what we are already doing.
We have a lot of capabilities in this organization.
Ben Watson and I could change jobs and handle them
without difficulty. We know what's going on in the
other departments and it wouldn't be any problem to
change them around. But this kind of change can't
help but put a halt on anything innovative.

Hayfield, too, felt that the holding pattern would deprive the
Victory organization of innovative thrusts at least for some time:

It seems that we have been able to go ahead with a lot
of routine changes, and there might still be innovation
in small ways in particular units. There will always
be changes going on, but the main hindrance of our
recent staffing difficulty has been that we haven't been
able to work hard on long-run, advance plans. But we
are keeping up each day.

The holding pattern, however, carried some undesirable consequences, such as continued uncertainty, restlessness, and, according to Nelling, management by crisis:

We can operate alright without filling the two vice
presidents' positions for a while. It hasn't always
mattered when there are vacancies there, because
we have a good staff. All the department heads are
very good. Sure there has been a lot of change. . . .
What happens is that everything piles up. Things go

along all right at first. The hospital kind of runs itself. We were so well organized that nothing much
happened for a while after Mr. Wright and the two
vice presidents left. However, when we go along
without filling those positions, we reach a stage of
putting out fires. It's management by crisis all the
time now. I'm handling one crisis after another and
things aren't getting any better.

THE NEW LEADER AT VICTORY

Robert Grepman, the new chief administrator for Victory
Hospital, was hired just two months prior to the appointment of
Norfield's new president. Grepman was careful and deliberate in
reviewing the organization's problems. An observer in Norfield
noted that the pace of activities increased, but they were slow in
returning to the level they had reached under Wright.
Wright had predicted that his successor would be a member
of the church denomination with which Victory was affiliated:

I am not a member of this hospital's church demonina-
tion, and I think I am the only administrator in the
whole system that isn't, at least in a top slot. I'm
more of a Presbyterian than anything else and actually, I'm a liberal. Being a liberal around here has
been an interesting experience. But I'll bet you'll
find that both in the case of Manton's permament re-
placcment and my own that they'll fill it with someone
from the hospital's denomination. Of course they say
it doesn't make any difference and that they are looking for the right man regardless, but you'll see that
he'll fit right in.

Wright was correct on all counts. Both Manton's successor
and his own were members of the hospital's donomination. Grepman
himself commented that:

I don't think the board of trustees would sacrifice
competence for religious affiliation. All other things
being equal, I know they prefer somebody who is of
this denomination in all key positions. It is not a
formal policy but it works out that way. One thing
I don't agree with though is the fact that our board
memberships are also restricted to this denomination.

> I think this is a detriment. We are a community hos-
> pital, and I think we should have a more representa-
> tive board. But I'm sure our hospital has not been
> hurt in any way by the emphasis on having adminis-
> trators from this denomination.

Grepman proved to be an able young administrator, modest, calm in temperament, and positive in outlook. He appeared to enjoy hard work and to recognize that he faced staffing problems. One was what to do about the two still-vacant vice presidential positions that had covered the main operating departments. He moved slowly on this, preferring careful study. The result was that department heads brought problems either to Grepman himself or to the other vice presidents, thus adding to their burden. These practices fed the internecine struggle for power and greatly intensified the administrative burdens for Grepman, Winters, and Nelling.

Nelling was not unduly perturbed by shifts in responsibilities at the vice presidential level. She welcomed the shift of functions from those of the departed vice presidents:

> Interviewer: Won't the loss of functions in the two
> operating groups make the two vice presidential
> vacancies less attractive to potential candidates?
> Nelling: It could be looked at that way. According to
> one theory, it would take some important things
> out of each of the vice presidents' list of functions.
> As a matter of fact, Bill Wright discussed the
> issue while he was still here. He wanted to keep
> the functions under the vice presidents to make
> them important jobs. But I don't think it's going
> to work that way necessarily. I don't see why the
> two vacancies cannot still be filled by very good
> people.

Nelling's observations did not match those reported earlier for Wright, who had said that he preferred to make periodic, temporary switches in the functional departments assigned to the vice presidents. And while both Ellis and Watson had reported that they were capable of handling any of the functions in either group, they had not been in their vice presidential posts very long and they resisted Wright's change impulses.

Shortly after his arrival, Grepman indicated that he was studying a reorganization of the department functions assigned to former vice presidents Ellis and Watson:

Interviewer: As they stood until now, the functions of
each vice president were rather evenly balanced?
Grepman: Yes, that's right. Heretofore there was an
effort to keep the two groups balanced as to important and unimportant functions. I think there's a
drawback to having these two groups equal. Actually, I'm a neophyte in this business. I've only
been in health care work six years. But during
that time my experience has been that wherever
you have two equal units like these there is trouble.
You can see what happened when the two men both
left suddenly. I think it is better to have one man
in a top slot and the other in kind of a training or
development position under that top person.

As matters turned out, however, Grepman replaced the two former
operating vice presidents, maintaining the two parallel units virtually intact. Over 18 months later it was observed by the researchers that there were no major structural changes in the organization
of Victory Hospital.

In sum, the Victory organization reacted extensively to changes
in the Norfield Organization. Victory's changes were traumatic in
their emotional impact on people. Changes in organizational staffing
substantially terminated or slowed other kinds of innovation and
change. A holding pattern emerged which protected the organization
but limited it to maintenance of the status quo. Victory thus successfully coped with externally and internally induced changes. We
turn now to a further analysis of the organizational context for innovation and change.

NOTES

1. Carl N. Platou and James A. Rice, "Multihospital Hold-
ing Companies," Harvard Business Review (May–June 1972): 14-20,
146-49. See also Montague Brown, "Contract Management: Latest
Development in the Trend towards Regionalization of Hospital and
Health Services," Hospital and Health Services Administration 21
(Winter 1976): 40-50; James P. Cooney and Thomas L. Alexander,
Multihospital Systems: An Evaluation (Evanston, Ill.: Health
Services Center of the Hospital Research and Educational Trust,
Northwestern University, 1975), 4 vols.; B. Jon Jaeger, ed.,
A Decade of Implementation: The Multiple Hospital Management
Concept Revisited (Durham, N.C.: Department of Health Adminis-
tration, Duke University, 1975); Montague Brown and Howard L.

Lewis, Hospital Management Systems: Multi-Unit Organization and Delivery of Health Care (Germantown, Md.: Aspen Systems Corporation, 1976).

2. Jeffrey Pfeffer and Gerald R. Salancik, "Organizational Context and the Characteristics and Tenure of Hospital Administrators," Academy of Management Journal 20 (April 1977): 47-88.

3

THE ORGANIZATIONAL CONTEXT OF
INNOVATION AND CHANGE

Innovation and change occur within two interacting frameworks: (1) the structural pattern of organization and associated managerial and administrative processes, and (2) the human capabilities for creativity, innovation, and change. This chapter analyzes the overall organizational context and the influence of lateral relationships on innovation and change. Figure 3.1 shows the parts of the basic model presented in Chapter 1 that are explored in this and the following chapters.

THE BUREAUCRATIC CONTEXT

The concept of bureaucracy includes two sets of contextual factors: (1) structure and (2) the administrative process, including management or leadership styles. The balance between the two sets of factors varies widely from one organization to another. Almost every organization displays some bureaucratic characteristics, but administrators can modify their nature and impact to achieve goals such as job satisfaction or innovation and change.

For purposes of comparison, it is useful to examine Weber's concept of bureaucracy as an "ideal type." This ideal type unites the structural and process sectors into a stable, ongoing system which includes a hierarchy of levels, fixed positions of authority and responsibility, planned succession to office, specific rules and firm discipline, strong reward and punishment systems, and the transcendence of positions over people. These elements are "ideal" for the pursuit of efficiency goals, and they lead to operating the bureaucracy as a closed system. That is, it is relatively rigid, and closed to all but the most necessary interactions with the environment. The

FIGURE 3.1

Partial Model Showing Organizational Elements
in Change and Innovation

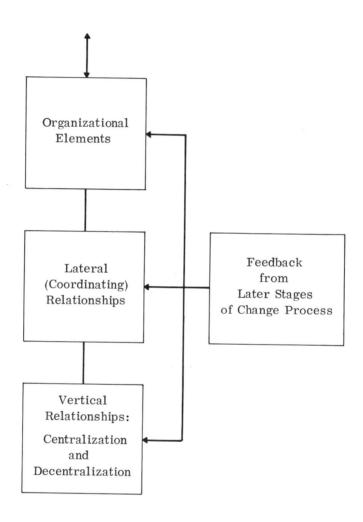

Source: Constructed by the author.

organization's outward postures are guarded and conservative. Autonomy and self-containment are idealized. It clings to self-preserving values and beliefs.[1]

In such a system, innovation and change are subservient to the forces of stability: the use of trained rather than natural leaders, the rigidity of procedures, the reverence of organization for its own sake, the tendency for adequate rather than optimum decisions, the use of merit systems to differentiate among members, and reliance on legalism in rule enforcement. Accordingly, innovations and changes that do occur are paced and controlled more by internal needs than by external forces. Change may even appear as deviant behavior—actions unsuccessfully restrained by policy and standard procedure. Managerial change and innovation tend to be gradual and are mainly defensive with respect to all but the most compelling outside forces.

Actual organizations can only approximate the ideal bureaucratic type. There is evidence to indicate that (1) the traditional model of bureaucracy, whatever its faults, is not so restrictive to innovation and change as has been widely supposed,[2] (2) managers can modify bureaucratic behavior to accommodate concerns beyond productive or economic efficiency,[3] and (3) advocates of the open system model argue successfully for modifications of, or alternatives to, bureaucracy.[4]

THE OPEN ORGANIZATION

The concepts of closed and open systems represent opposite poles on a continuum, with particular hospitals falling somewhere between the polar extremes. An organization is open to the extent that it is responsive to influences in its environment, oriented toward change and improvement, and flexible in its structure and administrative practice. Traditional structure is deemphasized. The open organization is sensitive to growth and development opportunities. It adapts skillfully to external influences, and copes aggressively with a turbulent environment. The more open the organization, the more sensitive it is to the needs and feelings of its members. According to Heydebrand, the hospital is responding to changes that lead to openness:

> If any organization is an example of how to survive between the need to routinize emergencies and the need to constantly improve and maximize the preservation of human values about life and health, it is the modern hospital. Therefore it is also one of the fastest changing organizations. . . .[5]

While hospitals display highly bureaucratic characteristics, they are moving toward more open systems. Shulz and Johnson assert that although there are still autocratic, bureaucratic managers schooled in Weberian bureaucracy, it became increasingly apparent in the 1960s that the hospital had to learn to deal more adequately with its external environment and that a behavioral systems model was necessary to incorporate this development.[6]

Demands from the public sector for improvement of services and for restraining rising costs put pressures on the hospital. This tests the bureaucracy's ability to respond to external realities. There is an inherent conflict between high demands for change from the external environment and the organization's need for bureaucratic stability and rational administration. Heydebrand expresses this dilemma cogently:

> While considerations of efficiency and economic rationality become increasingly dominant in today's hospital technology and management, they can never fully explain nor justify the always slightly precarious character of hospital operations, the constant adjustments to variable work loads, and the need to deal reasonably yet responsibly with uncertainty and critical situations.[7]

Pressures also impinge upon the bureaucratically organized hospital from such external sources as technological change or changes in other parts of the health care system, and from the demands of persons or groups claiming broad societal or cultural interests in society's health problems. These pressures reinforce the trend in hospitals to become more open. The hospital is a central focus for the very complex and increasingly sophisticated technology utilized by all the health care professions. This technology cuts in two opposite directions. On the one hand, it has led to what Kaluzny has referred to as the ascendancy of large, complex formal organizations typified by the Norfield multi-unit complex. But on the other hand, the hospital organization needs to adapt to changing environmental demands. At some point in its growth cycle, however, the increasingly sophisticated technology begins to project its own internally derived processes and requirements, making it desirable for the organization to be more selective and independent in its responses to sources of change.[8]

In any case, the studies at Victory indicate that external demands, such as those of technological change, are mediated through the hospital's own technological and professional employees, as well as members of the medical staff, and that the administrator's role is to adjudicate a balance between internal and external pressures for change.

OPENNESS VERSUS BUREAUCRACY AT VICTORY

Victory Hospital had a highly bureaucratic organizational design. However, the management styles of the top two echelons of managers were closer to those of the open organization than to those of bureaucracy. From the third echelon (department heads reporting to vice presidents) downward, the elements of bureaucracy in both structure and style were predominant.

Although the medical staff also had some bureaucratic features, it reflected even more the informal attitudes toward structural relationships and administration generally ascribed to open or adaptive systems and common among professionals. The flexible mechanisms for the medical staff included the use of short-tenure, elective positions for administration and a complex committee system which kept medical administration in a more fluid state. Physicians tended to regard administration and organization as a means to professional ends rather than ends in themselves.

The top echelons of administrators and the members of the medical staff viewed Victory Hospital as highly open to innovation and change, according to Wright:

> We are always open here about our activities. We like to share our situation here with others. We have a lot of interchange going on all the time. A lot of people come here to see what we are doing. . . . There have been more than twenty studies made around here on all types of problems during the past year. . . . We expect to gain a lot when an outsider like you comes in to make a study.

Wright viewed Victory as a highly innovative hospital. He had staffed it with energetic, creative people. He stated that the level of innovation was high compared to that in other hospitals he knew, but acknowledged that factors such as location or type of hospital might be important: "I have a habit of measuring everything around here on a ten-point scale. If we measure innovation on a ten-point scale, I would say that our organization rates seven or eight."

The two operations vice presidents shared these perceptions of openness. According to Ellis, "We are very open to ideas here." And Ben Watson stated that:

> The system here is open enough. The quickest way to
> shut off change is not to see the department heads. I
> feel that I must be very accessible to them. I think
> everybody should get a hearing around here. We
> should at least talk to people when they have some-
> thing on their mind.

Watson attributed the open organizational climate to Wright's leadership: "Our administrator has developed a good climate here for
innovation and change. He is receptive to any idea within reason,
if we have evidence to support it. The environment here really
encourages innovation and change."

The belief that the organization was relatively open was also
apparent among members of the medical staff. According to one
physician, a past chief-of-staff:

> This hospital is highly innovative. We have very re-
> sponsive administrators. They are very able, and
> extremely willing to listen to our ideas and requests.
> I feel able to call anyone up at any time. I can call
> the administrator or any member of the board of
> trustees or our executive committee of the medical
> staff. We'll always get a quick hearing if we need it.

The hospital's chaplain and counselor, Al McBride, also
thought the Victory organization was highly innovative, attributing
great importance to openness at the top: "The main thing is to be
open to change. You can't wait around for permission from the
top. The top has to be open, to allow feedback and to let innovation
rise to the top." And further, he cited the importance of leadership:

> I don't think creativity is possible in a hostile, tight,
> and heavily bureaucratic syste. You can't be laissez-
> faire but confidence in people is necessary and also an
> awareness of their potential. It's something like
> Theory X versus Theory Y. You get more out of
> Theory Y. The key to it all is leadership, although
> some action is important too.

FLEXIBILITY

The open-system trait of flexibility or adaptiveness serves a
twofold function: (1) it enables the organization to cope with the
pressures of external change, and (2) it facilitates internal changes

that arise from the organization's needs as well as from external pressures. At Victory there was ample evidence that, though the hierarchy retained its essential form, substantial flexibility of structure existed at the top. For example, Wright did not regard the assignments of responsibilities and departments to the two operations vice presidents as fixed:

> As to the functions assigned to the operations vice presidents, there isn't any particular logic and we change them around from time to time. I believe that the assignment of departments to the vice presidents is for the purpose of training them rather than just having them run things. The fact that there is overlap and a frequent change of boss for the department heads helps to train the vice presidents they report to, as well as the department heads themselves.

Further flexibility came from Wright's conferral of decision-making authority upon Watson and Ellis equal to his own. In addition to Wright's being on call at all times, Watson and Ellis were also on call, especially on weekends. They could make any overall decision affecting Victory at any time Wright was not available. There was also a strong belief in reducing the rigidity of reporting relationships. The idea of "bosses" was played down both at the top and at middle-management levels, especially by Wright.

At a lower level, a nursing supervisor described herself as an "assistant to" the four patient education specialists she supervised, rather than as a boss:

> These specialists were here long before I came. They reported directly to the director of nursing. Now they report to me. I say they report to me, but don't be misled. I don't feel like I'm their boss. Mostly I'm their assistant, or an administrative arm. The assistant director for staff education also has a lot of influence with them and therefore you can't really say that I'm their boss.

It is possible that these verbalized perceptions of openness and flexibility are mere postures. Yet the nursing vice president was released six months after the new administrator came aboard, allegedly because of her autocratic and overbearing manner. A nurse confirmed that she functioned the opposite of the way she talked, and ran to the chief administrator with everything she learned from subordinates. There was clearly a climate of openness cultivated at the top and desired for the organization as a whole. Those whose behavior did not fit this mode were ostracized.

Let us now examine in more detail the structural context, including departmentalization, interdepartmental relations, and the presence of organizational slack.

STRUCTURAL FACTORS

Veney and Kahn indicate that most researchers have stressed the characteristics of organization members as the predominant causal variable in innovation and change. Nonpersonal variables, such as the physical or structural context of the organization, have been largely regarded as endogenous and hence not germane to the study of change. Their own study of the development of hospital service programs concluded that the elaboration of structure within a hospital is primarily a function of context and structure but that a smaller independent force is a function of the context and the chief administrator.[9]

Researchers have also examined such variables as organizational size, resources, and control as influences on innovation. Hage and Aiken found in studying health and welfare agencies that the implementation of innovations was related to organizational complexity.[10] Mytinger[11] and Palumbo[12] both found positive correlations among organizational size, resources, and implementation. Several researchers have examined community variables such as urbanization in relation to program implementation.

Victory hospital clearly met a number of contextual conditions favoring innovative change: large size, complex (multi-unit) structure, an urban setting, and a relatively open system by which it is attuned to environmental pressures and internal flexibility. We will now examine departmental structures and selected managerial functions as they related to innovation and change processes at Victory. The vertical dimensions of organization will be considered in the following chapter.

The Impact of Departmentalization

A key structural element in bureaucracy is its horizontal differentiation into functional and other types of specialized units, with associated problems of communication, coordination, and articulation. Innovations and changes frequently cut across departmental lines, and they therefore serve either as integrative or divisive forces. Except for minor internal changes, a change in

one unit usually has major impacts on other units. As one of the
operations vice presidents stated:

> Hospitals can be very innovative. In fact, a hospital
> has more opportunity to be innovative than a business.
> In hospitals there are so many problems to solve, so
> many things happening all at once. Therefore, the
> need for innovation is much greater. Innovation can
> happen in any department.

By viewing the hospital organization as a system, one can
treat analytically the impacts of a change in one subsystem or in
one or more of the other subsystems. A good example is found in
the data processing department which must react to every change
that affects information processing. Thus it serves as a monitoring
and control center for a vast sector of change. According to the
head of data processing, flexibility is important:

> We're constantly changing because of our interaction
> with other departments when we come up with new
> methods of recording and processing information. I
> have to take a different approach with every personality
> in the hospital. Usually, it's changes in procedures
> that affect us the most. We have to come up with a new
> reporting system whenever there is a change in pro-
> cedure and this happens a lot in our hospital. There-
> fore we have to be flexible and ready to accept new
> reporting systems. For example, pharmacy changes
> its reporting system often, because it is always dis-
> pensing new medications. We don't find out about it
> until we get the charges for them. Then we have to be
> ready to respond.

How structural changes affect data processing is illustrated
by the creation of a new department of ostomy therapy. The data
processing department had to monitor cost and revenue information,
because the new department head needed data with which to justify
her job.

The data processing department, while it necessarily must
react to changes in other departments or to new departments, also
initiates changes designed to improve efficiency and coordination of
information processing. According to the department head:

> I interact with the old and new departments by giving
> them advice on handling patient charges and improving

the efficiency of their departments. My department sees
a problem before any other department in the hospital.
Therefore, it's our responsibility to make sure that this
record function runs smoothly. For example, radiology
had three people working on patient charges who were
uncoordinated in that they were all assigning different
patient numbers. This was inefficient and the computer
couldn't handle all those numbers because of the forms
and therefore they were having to do extra work. All I
did was inform them that they needed to become coordinated and offer some suggestions on how they could handle
their patient charges better. . . . The Emergency Room
is another example of inefficiency in record-keeping
skills. There is a lack of coordination, and the people
who run Emergency are medically oriented as opposed
to a business orientation. I raised a little flak with
higher administration a while back because they weren't
coordinated. When we started sending them revenue
reports based on what they were sending us, the director
of the Emergency Room could see what had to be done.

The cardiovascular laboratory also reflected the impact on
its work of changes in other departments. Here the bulk of the
changes stopped short of innovation, but the laboratory manager
perceived that technical change often derives from managerial
policies and the need for cost-effective procedures:

Any change in the hospital that affects patient care
is going to affect our department indirectly. Actually, there is little direct effect that a department
will have on the lab except to make more work for us.
For instance, nursing may set up a new intensive
care unit. This is going to mean more work in the
hemodynamic monitoring of the patient but is not
going to make us any more innovative. . . . As a
matter of fact, most of the innovation . . . is more or
less a result of policies and guidelines that the cardiovascular lab has established. Take, for instance,
how the maintenance department a few years ago developed an inexpensive method for keeping water cool
for our heart pump machine. All we told them is that
we wanted the water at a constant temperature and
they took it from there. I know that we sometimes
cause problems for other departments, but we always
do it with the motive of improving patient care and
not necessarily for our own benefit.

An example of problems in the allocation of tasks and responsibilities among departments was found in the case of the neurosciences laboratory. EKG work was once in this department, but it
had been transferred to the cardiovascular laboratory. This altered
budgetary matters in both departments, since EKG work was regarded as profitable whereas the rest of the department's responsibilities were not. According to the head of neurosciences:

> Neuroscience is commonly not a profitable depart-
> ment in most hospitals. As a matter of fact, we've
> never broken even in our department. Most hospitals
> will put EKG with their neuroscience department just
> to make it a profitable department.

Interdepartmental Conflict

Changes made by one department of the hospital not only led to
changes in other departments as they adjusted to the demands of
interdependency. They also engendered conflicting sentiments and
reactions. In Victory, these were met by management postures
emphasizing communication, coordination, and planning. Thus
certain management functions are brought to bear to soften the
potentially disruptive effects of change. Conflict also absorbs
energies that might otherwise go into innovation and change.
Physical conditions were often sources of conflict. In neurosciences, role and status conflicts among technicians arose from
their placement in the medical laboratory instead of having their
own private space. According to the head of neurosciences:

> The most important thing to make our department
> more efficient would be to give us a better loca-
> tion . . . we do a lot of out-patient work, but be-
> cause we are in the back of the lab, it is difficult for
> patients to find us. Although we are not a part of
> the lab, we are in their space, and some of their
> policies are different from ours. . . . The tech-
> nicians in neurosciences understand, yet they
> resent being classed as part of the medical labora-
> tory. I'm not saying we don't get along with them.
> We do. But I think our department deserves more
> autonomy.

Laboratory units provided a center of both conflict and cooperation because of functional interdependencies. For example, the

radiological laboratory, like data processing, has linkages with
numerous other units. According to the chief technician, cooperation is important:

> Radiology ties in with all the departments, but particu-
> larly with nursing services. We work hard to get and
> keep their cooperation. We try to avoid technical
> squabbles with the nurses on the floor. I don't mean
> we have to do any bootlicking or anything like that
> but it is a good idea to get along with them if we can.

Often the desire to cooperate is not sufficient, and conflict
leads to invoking higher authority. In the case of conflicts between
radiology and nursing, the chief technician took the problem of
nurses failing to provide transportation of patients to the laboratory
to Wright:

> He came down at 6:30 in the afternoon to catch the
> beginning of the night shift and see how things were
> working. I knew that he would help us. . . . We get
> along pretty well with the nurses but on this problem
> of transport, one of the nurses told one of my tech-
> nicians that the nurses had voted to cancel all trans-
> port service. That was a silly vote. When I told the
> vice president of nursing about it, I said "What if
> I gave orders to cancel all x-rays for the patients?"
> She said that she thought they were going by the
> rules, but that "rules were made to be bent" and we
> should cooperate.

Further evidence of organizational conflict was also found between the radiology department and the nursing staff, but here, too,
conscious coordination was preferred to going to the vice president.
According to the chief radiological technician:

> We try to get along with the nurses. Neither side just
> runs to the administrator over any old thing. We might
> talk to Mr. Ellis but first we try to solve our problems
> in our own way. The administrators like it better that
> way too.

In the case of the medical staff, there was also evidence that
coordination was often achieved by appeal to higher authority. Traditionally, there is a pronounced cleavage between the medical staff
group and administrative personnel. This hiatus is analyzed as role

conflict in Chapter 11, but here it is important to note that at
Victory, committees fulfill a mediating role that supports innovation and change:

> Interviewer: What do you do if you have trouble estab-
> lishing a new practice or procedure?
> Physician: What happens is that problems go first to the
> executive committee of the medical staff. The medi-
> cal staff always tries to work out its own problems.
> Everything is thoroughly discussed and in most cases
> by the time we do that we have the answers. The
> administrators sound every one out and when they
> hear no objections, they generally go ahead. But if
> something is blocked, we have a connection to the
> board of trustees because the chairman of the medical
> staff's executive committee is on the board.

The functions of coordination and integration of contentions
over change require firm control at the top. Wright insisted upon
control procedures which provided him with a continuous picture of
ongoing activities, so that problems arising from change could be
coordinated. The elaborate systems of record keeping, data processing, and reports that pervaded Victory Hospital were highly
bureaucratic, but they were rationalized by the belief that they were
necessary for control as well as for planning and change. Wright
commented that:

> A lot of people complain because they have to submit monthly
> reports. They don't do that in the rest of the Norfield or-
> ganization. I'm the only one that gets reports like this. But
> it's necessary to keep track of what is going on. Sure, with-
> out the reports I would still know a lot, but I wouldn't be able
> to see what the changes were, what our progress is, how
> people are coming along. And I might fail to see something
> important if it isn't down in writing. This is an organized
> way to proceed and I think people are getting used to it now.

The multi-unit design of the Norfield Medical Complex also
posed problems of communication, coordination, and control. But
the Norfield central officers gave momentum to planning at Victory.
Ellis explained how planning for setting objectives paves the way for
innovation:

> Our whole Norfield organization is unique. It's a new
> concept. We have problems of structure, geography,

and logistics. This means there is an absence of face-
to-face communication. When you have differences in
objectives, that's a complication. But if we can get
together and work out our objectives, we are in a position to go ahead with innovation. If individuals are
good, if you can understand their survival motivations,
and if the people know what a good job is so it can be
evaluated, then you can drive ahead. Take myself,
for example. I find there is very little overlap between
me and my counterparts, or with Mr. Wright, because
we can talk about our problems.

One interesting type of organizational change was forced upon
Victory by the central office group in order to improve coordination
and communication. Leonard Hayfield, vice president of finance at
Norfield, initiated the appointment of a vice president for business
administration at Victory. According to Wright,

It was Len Hayfield's idea. A lot of our decisions are
based on personality, not structure. We build our
organization around people. Len felt we needed this
position for rapport between the Norfield and Victory
organizations. He instructed me to hire an accountant
to be called vice president for business administration.

Nelling was the first occupant of this new position. She gave
the following account, reflecting on reporting to two superiors:

Interviewer: The idea seems to have taken quite a
while to be worked out.
Nelling: Yes. Things don't happen as suddenly as they
seem to on the surface. It takes a lot of work to
get ready to make a change like that.
Interviewer: And why do you think the position was
created?
Nelling: It evolved as an interface between Victory
Hospital and the central office. I report directly to
Mr. Wright, although I also report to Mr. Hayfield
in the central office. This double reporting doesn't
cause me any problems. In fact, it was Len's concept that I would report primarily to Mr. Wright.
Actually, I operate in both worlds, the world of
finance and computers, and also the world of administrative problems, putting out fires, watching the
pickets, and things like that. The whole idea came

about because Central Administration had goals
that didn't quite coincide with our activities in the
hospital. It was a way of linking them together and
providing better communication.

In Victory itself, however, one mechanism for planning, coordinating, and controlling, as well as for innovation and change,
existed only minimally: the use of departments organized on a staff
basis. Activities that are staff functions in many organizations were
handled by the line units themselves. Victory had a personnel office
and a public relations director, but these functions were directed
primarily from the headquarters organization. They were minimal
in scope and their directors served mainly as links to the central
office. The personnel function at Victory was largely clerical.

Organizational Slack

Successful records of innovation are mainly found in organizations that are very different from the tight organization system of
the bureaucracy. But the one thing that a bureaucracy can have
that facilitates innovation is organizational resources. The term
organizational slack refers to the fact that the organization's
achievement level has been greater than its aspiration level. [13]
Slack results when an accumulation of resources occurs because
the organization is able to achieve its objectives with less expendi-
ture of resources than projected. As a result, resources are
available for allocation to subgroup or individual goals, including
those of change and innovation. [14]
Organizational slack represents a relative degree of organizational affluence. It consists of uncommitted resources—flexibilities
with respect to people, money, materials, and the like. Exactly
how slack increases innovation is not well understood but the fact
that it does so is apparent. It has been suggested that unused resources are perhaps an embarrassment to the administrator, leading to a search for something to do with them. A use must be found
for them because they are there. Also slack increases the disposition to engage in riskier actions for higher stakes than is true of
administrators with few resources at their disposal.
In analyzing the consequences of organizational slack, March
and Simon found that unlimited resources tend to decrease the demand for joint decision making, and to increase the differentiation
of goals. Organization slack also reduced intergroup conflict within
organizations by eliminating the need to resolve contending subgroup differentiation. When slack fades and resources become
scarce, intergroup competition increases. [15]

Wilson suggests that organizations with a scarcity of resources tend to suppress conflict, maintain hierarchical controls, and emphasize explicit organizational goals. More affluent organizations tend to avoid conflict, relax hierarchical controls, develop new products and services, and engage in the elaboration of imaginative but vaguely defined goals. Wilson has also raised the problem of whether innovation is accounted for by the devil theory or the necessity theory. That is, "the devil makes work for idle hands," or "necessity is the mother of invention." Wilson writes:

> The devil theory of innovation was devised . . . because the necessity theory was not supported by the facts. Being on the ragged edge of adversity did not appear to make firms more inventive or more adaptive; on the contrary, the prosperous firms seemed more willing to try new ideas. A theory was obviously necessary to show why successful firms innovated; if this could be done without abandoning the previous theory—most unsuccessful firms innovated also, but in a different way—so much the better. Necessity and the devil could be brought into a fruitful partnership.[16]

The devil theory, implying the presence of organization slack, is supported by the research at Victory, which was successful and prosperous. Yet it experienced adversity too. Crises such as labor strife and severe top management turnover temporarily slowed innovation and change, yet produced an amalgamation of interests and a camaraderie among remaining managers as shoulders were put to the wheel. Necessity too produced change, but it was change directed at survival of the system rather than the advancement of it.

The analysis of organization slack in relation to innovation raises the question of the legitimacy of goals, which is to say, the intentions of "owners." The "owners'" values are not necessarily advanced by innovation, particularly the riskier varieties. They may therefore view the generation of slack as contrary to their interests. We can now observe that the replacement of top managers at Norfield and Victory with managers far more conservative than their predecessors manifested the intent to curb innovative, risky growth. Two pieces of evidence reinforce this view. First, the unionization drive represented pressure for a greater cut of the affluence melon demanded by the workers. Therefore, too much slack caused problems. The cost of restraining unionism thus included the reduction of slack and hence of innovation. Second, the already conservative managers at Bright Hospital were relatively unaffected by the chain resignation traumas at Norfield and Victory.

It is ironic that slack appears to have been viewed by Norfield's board of trustees as causing organizational stress, since slack is also needed to combat stress. The trade-off for reducing stress is to risk a reduction in innovation.[17]

PROGRAMMATIC INNOVATION

Where there is little or no organization slack and an organization is busy managing existing programs, initiation of new programs will be slow. But when a new program is developed, a new structural unit is often created to carry out the new program. Thus, innovating activities of a programmatic nature tend to occur in spurts of energy and activities, which become established firmly in the bureaucracy. During the first stage of planning and preparation, there is a period of excitement for the people involved. Those committed to it may put in overtime, enjoying the challenge and the change. They display feelings of pride and pleasure in their work. The transition to programmed status results in routinizing matters so that the excitement fades and feelings of anticlimax set in. Thus, there is a continuous need for generating new programs that are relatively unhampered by tradition and precedent, to provide challenging, stimulating experiences for the members of an organization.[18]

The traits and capabilities of managers needed in the innovating phase differ from those needed in the program execution stage. The former requires idea people; the latter fares better under orderly bureaucrats. Clearly, the hospital needs an appropriate mix of stabilizers and innovators, with adequate recognition given to both types. Programs help because they identify innovative ideas and provide for experiment and the development of the necessary operating mechanisms. The danger is that, once established, programs may lose their excitement as innovations become rigidly locked into the machinery of the bureaucracy.[19]

We turn next to an analysis of how the vertical dimension of organization structure influences the processes of innovation and change.

NOTES

1. Max Weber, Essays in Sociology (New York: Oxford University Press, 1946). See also Peter M. Blau, Bureaucracy in Modern Society (New York: Random House, 1956); Ralph H. Hummel, The Bureaucratic Experience (New York: St. Martin's Press, 1977).

2. See, for example, Arthur L. Stinchcombe, Creating Efficient Industrial Administration (New York: Academic Press, 1974). Stinchcombe's findings on innovation in three South American steel plants are at considerable variance with common presuppositions about the bureaucracy's inhibiting effects on innovation.

3. See, for example, John G. Maurer, ed., Readings in Organization Theory: Open Systems Approaches (New York: Random House, 1971).

4. Ibid. See also Warren G. Bennis, American Bureaucracy (New Brunswick, N.J.: Transaction Books, 1970), and Warren G. Bennis, The Unconscious Conspiracy: Why Leaders Can't Lead (New York: AMACOM, 1976).

5. Wolf Heydebrand, Hospital Bureaucracy: A Comparative Study of Organizations (New York: Dunellen Press, 1973), pp. xxvii-xxix.

6. Rockwell Shulz and Alton C. Johnson, Management of Hospitals (New York: McGraw-Hill, 1976), pp. 33-42. See also Duncan Neuhauser, "The Hospital as a Matrix Organization," Hospital Administration, Fall 1972, pp. 8-25.

7. Heydebrand, op. cit., p. xxix.

8. Arnold D. Kaluzny, "Innovation in Health Services: Theoretical Framework and Review of Research," Health Services Research, Summer 1974, pp. 104-05.

9. James E. Veney and Jahanger Kahn, "Causal Paths in the Elaboration of Organizational Structure: A Case of Hospital Services," Health Services Research, Summer 1973, pp. 139-50.

10. J. Hage and M. Aiken, "Program Change and Organizational Properties: A Comparative Analysis," American Journal of Sociology 72, no. 503 (March 1967).

11. R. E. Mytinger, "Innovation in Local Health Services," PHS Publication no. 1664-2 (Washington, D.C.: U.S. Government Printing Office, 1968).

12. D. Palumbo et al., "A Systems Analysis of Local Public Health Departments," paper presented at the 95th Annual Meeting of the American Public Health Association, Miami, Fla., October 1967.

13. Thompson, op. cit., pp. 34-35, 43-46.

14. James G. March and Herbert A. Simon, Organizations (New York: Wiley, 1958), pp. 126-27.

15. Ibid. See also Kenneth E. Knight, "A Descriptive Model of the Intra-Firm Innovation Process," Journal of Business 40, no. 4 (October 1967): 478-96; and Mohr, op. cit., p. 119.

16. James Q. Wilson, "Necessity vs. the Devil," in Bennis, op. cit., pp. 157-60.

17. Thompson, op. cit., pp. 44-46.

18. March and Simon, op. cit., p. 187. See also Frederick C. Dyer and John M. Dyer, Bureaucracy vs. Creativity (Miami: University of Miami Press, 1969), Ch. 4.

19. See Jerald Hage and M. Aiken, "Program Change and Organizational Properties," American Journal of Sociology 72 (March 1967): 503-19; Jerald Hage, "A Systems Perspective in Organization Change," in Innovations in Health Care Organizations, ed. Arnold D. Kaluzny et al. (Chapel Hill: School of Public Health, University of North Carolina, 1974); and Jerald Hage and R. Dewar, "The Prediction of Organization Performance: The Case of Program Innovation," Administrative Science Quarterly 18 (September 1973): 279-90.

4

LEVELS OF INNOVATION AND CHANGE:

CENTRALIZATION AND DECENTRALIZATION

To the extent that an organization is bureaucratic, it consists of a system that distributes formal power and authority vertically in a series of gradations known as the hierarchy. At the top are the persons and positions of greatest authority; by delegation, authority is more and more restricted in scope as one moves down the hierarchy. We saw in the previous chapter that Victory Hospital was largely a bureaucracy but that, while structures and management practices were in the main appropriate to a bureaucracy, attitudes and perceptions of the open organization were present among the top two levels of administrators. At lower levels, however, bureaucratic tendencies remained predominant, this in spite of the fact that the top administrators at Victory effectively communicated their attitudes and perceptions of openness to the units below. We will now examine how the processes of centralization and decentralization affected innovation and change in Victory Hospital. Figure 4.1 depicts the relevant part of the model under discussion.

The extent to which authority is assigned to successively lower levels can be depicted as a continuum whose poles are centralization and decentralization. Centralization is here defined as the extent to which power and authority are concentrated in the top positions of the hospital. Decentralization is defined as the extent of autonomy resulting from the downward dispersion of authority by delegation.

The research literature on innovation views the decentralization-innovation relationship mainly from a global perspective. That is, open (organic) organizations are found to be innovative, and the decentralization implicit in the open organization is a primary predictor of innovation. But the literature also indicates that decentralization has a differential effect on the various stages of the

FIGURE 4.1

Partial Model Showing Relationship of Vertical Structure
to Human Capabilities, Ideation, and Expectations

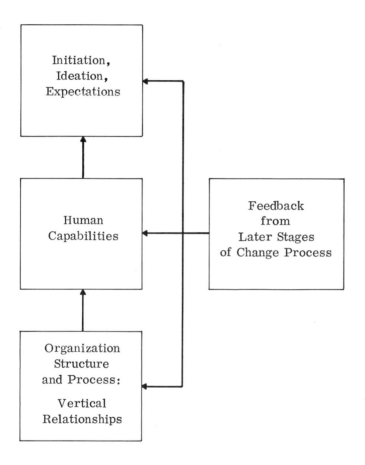

Source: Constructed by the author.

model presented in Chapter 1. In open organizations, decentralization increases initiation activity by less restrictive communications and greater autonomy of work units and individuals. The participants of the open organization generate greater ego involvement and commitment that facilitate the implementation stage and improve the acceptance of change.[1]

Pierce and Delbecq, based on a review of the literature, provide the following proposition:

> Decentralization will be positively related with initiation and implementation, there will be a stronger positive relation for initiation than implementation, and both will be more positive than adoption. Adoption may, in fact, be negatively related to innovation.[2]

This proposition cannot be fully evaluated until we have discussed the processes of initiation, implementation, and adoption in later chapters. In this chapter, we shall make a preliminary assessment of the proposition and consider the conditions precedent to the proposition by analyzing the influences of centralization and decentralization on innovation and change.

VICTORY AND THE CENTRAL OFFICE

The multi-unit structure of the Norfield Medical Complex is itself an innovation in the hospital field, and in the nation as a whole this type of structure is increasing. Today, nearly 15 percent of the nation's hospitals are members of multisystem complexes. In 1973, only 350 such systems existed, but it has been suggested that by 1983 most general hospitals will be members of integrated systems.[3]

The administrative group in the Norfield office provided an additional force for centralization that a single-unit institution would not have. Thompson traces the need for increasing centralization to two general causes: (1) the personal needs of persons in positions of power and (2) technical development. Both causes were evident in the Norfield-Victory relationship.[4]

The centralization of administrative control over finance, personnel administration, planning, overall policy, and purchasing in the Norfield headquarters thereby lessened the concern for these matters that would otherwise have been necessary in Victory. At the same time, the ability to control the administration of these matters relieved Norfield managers of anxieties that would result from having to predict the actions of Victory's managers. While this situation enhanced the power of managers within the Norfield offices and met their personal needs for control, it produced frustrations in Victory where actions and procedures had to conform to central requirements.

The technical causes also increased the tendency toward centralization. The central staff planned and reviewed capital expenditures and equipment purchases with the aim of assuring full utilization of resources and economic justifications of expenditures. The central group could mandate sharing between Bright and Victory. For example, central drug stocks were shared by a courier system with a truck making daily eight-mile runs between them.

In a centralized system of this type, according to Thompson, only those with authority at the center can legitimately innovate. The anxiety of central decision makers can be managed or reduced by enforcing conformity, thereby increasing the certainty and predictability of performance. But innovation is the by-product of freedom that gives individuals a sense of personal security so that they are not afraid to make choices, to do something new or different that is not dictated by authority, tradition, or personality. [5]

For several reasons this paradox was not entirely characteristic of the Norfield-Victory relationship. Norfield administrators maintained a low profile of minimal intrusion into Victory's operations. They viewed themselves as relating mainly to future plans for expansion, to improving community relations, to fund raising, and to influencing state and national legislation. Thus, they were oriented more to external affairs than to internal operations of the units. Also, they deliberately stressed the importance of autonomy of the hospital units, and conformity did not appear to be an issue between them. Procedural conformity was routine, but policy conformity was negotiable.

The significance of all this for innovation is that Norfield's centralization did not include strong control or influence over innovative behavior within Victory. An example is provided in the relationship between staff functions at Victory and those in the Norfield office.

STAFF GROUPS

Early in this study it was hypothesized that staff groups would be, as they traditionally are, a strong motivating influence for innovation and change. In the Norfield organization, however, this concept could not be supported. The reasons were twofold: (1) the staff groups were concentrated in the central office and (2) they emphasized service and control functions rather than innovation and change.

At Victory, all traditional staff functions had only rudimentary structures, since the bulk of the staff functions were located in the central office. For example, personnel functions were minimal and routine, with a small personnel staff under the line control of the director of personnel in the Norfield office.

The lack of a strong, organization-wide personnel program designed to capitalize on the human capabilities and potentials greatly inhibited innovation and change. In effect, the personnel management system within Victory was decentralized and informal. There were no central personnel policy manuals or handbooks for distribution to new or existing employees, although some department heads had written their own. In the absence of a strong, central personnel office staffed with professional personnel specialists, the separate units were doing their own recruiting, placing, and training of employees. Therefore, methods, practices, and policies differed substantially among the various units. Those units with highly professional or highly technical employees managed quite well, since access to sources of supply was possible through word-of-mouth communication by existing staff members and through contacts with schools and professional associations.

The role of the personnel office at Victory was essentially to process the paper work that resulted from the personnel efforts of the various organizational units. It was headed by a woman whose title was assistant personnel director and she had a counterpart at Bright Hospital. These two persons reported to a personnel director located in Norfield's central office. The assistant personnel director at Victory had one subordinate, an interviewer.

The central personnel office at Norfield was not a strong one, nor was it completely staffed or well organized. It was headed by a personnel director who in the second year of this study transferred to Victory as a research specialist and then resigned shortly thereafter. He was replaced in the Norfield office by the wage and salary administrator, on an acting basis. He had not been reporting to the personnel director, but was organized parallel to him. There were no specialists in selection, training, or labor relations, and no systematic work was done on such problems as morale, motivation, human relations, or manpower planning. The acting personnel director in Norfield continued also to perform his wage and salary functions. He had been at Norfield for only a year prior to these changes, and had an industrial rather than a hospital background.

This description of the structure and operations of the personnel functions at Norfield and Victory is not strikingly different from those that exist in many hospitals. What is significant is that such conditions provide only the most routine handling of personnel matters, and no resources are provided for accentuating organization-

wide employee development programs. Since morale and motivation are associated with high rates of innovation and change, the
organization loses an opportunity to benefit from the human capabilities present or potentially available.

Victory was receiving little or no guidance, direction, leadership, or coordination from Norfield in personnel matters. Nor were
the managers in Victory benefiting from central direction and guidance within Victory itself, as there were no professional personnel
managers. Therefore, at both levels the organizations involved
were not prepared to deal with unusual demands or peculiar, nonroutine events thrust upon them from the external environment.
The labor strife detailed earlier in this book is illustrative.

The central group at Norfield, through its line management
approach, could substantially influence innovation and change at
Victory. However, our observations indicated that apart from
major organizational changes, the central office was not a strong
force for innovation at Victory. It could, however, slow down the
processes of innovation and change while undergoing traumatic organizational changes of its own. In the previous chapter, it was
shown that when key officials left the central office (the president
and the personnel director), managers at Victory felt that maintenance of stability and the status quo, rather than innovation and
change, became their principal preoccupations.

According to Wright, line authority characterized all the
"staff" functions in the central office, not merely the personnel
function:

> In the central office, we have an executive committee
> composed of the key people in the central office and
> the administrators of Victory and Bright. The odd
> part is that it does not include any of the vice presi-
> dents or department heads from the hospitals. They
> have no voice in what happens. Remember that those
> people in the central office are all staff. So this com-
> mittee passes on actions and rules and regulations
> that the rest of us have to carry out in the hospitals.
> What you have is the staff giving orders to the line.
> That's contrary to anything I know about in the field
> of management.

Since the central staff groups functioned more in a line capacity than in the traditional staff roles of planning, advising, and
stimulating change, and since their counterpart functions in Victory
were minimal and subsidiary to the central groups, Victory was deprived of a strong motivating force for innovation and change. Since

innovation and change were found to be relatively high at Victory, it can be concluded that it is primarily the chief administrator and his vice presidents that provided the principal motivating influences for innovation and change. This was confirmed by the vice president for business operations at Victory:

> Interviewer: Do you think Victory and Bright differ in any substantial way as to their creativity and innovation?
>
> Nelling: (Smiling) It all depends on the administrator. Mr. Wright is an outstanding, creative, and innovative person. He's bound to inspire innovation and creativity throughout the organization. The administrator at Bright takes an entirely different point of view when it comes to initiating things. Definitely everyone agrees that Victory is better than Bright with respect to innovation. But, again, what is an innovation to one person might be a stupid idea to another. Bright is an excellent place. . . . It can still be good even though the innovation patterns are different.

PLANNING

It might be thought that the presence of a strong central office group would provide Victory's managers with strong leadership for planning and the determination of objectives. Such was not the case, however. The best resource was the personal capability and enthusiasm of Norfield's president, Robert Manton. But Manton was a strong believer in delegation and in addition was heavily engaged in relations with outside groups throughout the community and the nation. From Victory's point of view, according to Wright, there were no specific goals at the top. Victory therefore had to develop its own goals.

Victory's success at innovation and change accordingly depended heavily on its internal resources, principally its leadership. This in turn led to problems of time and work flow. If the central staff is not actively involved in planning, the time and work burdens press upon the internal organization. Another problem in planning is the fact that hospital production and work flow are determined largely by other people, chiefly patients or their physicians. The hospital has to have all its procedures and operations ready to go upon demand. In such a system the demands are hard to forecast.

According to Vice President Ellis, the rationing of a manager's time is a critical factor in innovation:

> If you have an easy operation, with stability and pre-
> dictability, you have a greater ability to innovate. If
> you have a fire-fighting operation, you can't even make
> any change at all, much less progress or innovate. If
> you have a clean day-to-day operation and people have
> time to think, it would be a strong motivator for inno-
> vation. . . . You're never going to get time for inno-
> vation under battle conditions. However, I think it is
> important to have good staff planners. That way you
> are paying some people to take the time. The way my
> job is running now, it's hard for me to find even an
> hour or so just to go away and think and let ideas
> come into my head.

IMPACT OF THE COMPUTER

Planning was greatly facilitated in Victory with the advent of
a new computer. However, this also strengthened the control fuhc-
tions of the central office and diminished the data processing responsibilities of other parts of the Victory organization. (Norfield's centralized computer service was at first physically located
at Bright Hospital, but controlled and operated by a consulting firm.
In 1974, however, the computer equipment was moved to the central office building.)

The computer was used for a number of purposes, including
general data processing and payrolls. It was also used by the admitting department for forecasting the admitting and patient census
and for staffing reports. For example, in admitting, the director
reported that:

> Forecasting is one of admitting's primary duties here.
> When we admit a patient, we send all the information
> to Bright by Telex. . . . The printout they send us
> each morning tells us what our census is, but it
> doesn't really make any predictions. I predict a
> month ahead or more what our census will be on the
> basis of what it has been and what I feel the trend is.
> Of course, I'm not always right, sometimes I'm not
> even close; however, a lot of times I'm within 1 or
> 2 percent. Hospital admissions is by nature un-
> predictable in that no one can really predict or ex-

plain the variations in patient census from one
day to another.

A unit coordinator of nursing reported the use of the computer in staffing:

> One of my primary responsibilities is to make sure that
> accurate up-to-date time schedules for staffing is
> maintained. . . . Until a few years ago I did this my-
> self but now central staffing makes out all our sched-
> ules six weeks at a time. It seems to work well.
> What happens is that they will have a statistical re-
> port of how many people we have on the floor on a
> full- or part-time basis. Then they come up with a
> schedule for us and send it to the floor. When we
> receive the schedule, we evaluate it and if we feel
> that it is correct, we send it back to central staff-
> ing with our approval. The only problem is when
> we're short of people. . . . Of course, any other
> scheduling system would probably have the same
> deficiency.

Purchasing was another major function centralized with computerization in the headquarters office. Most managers at Victory
recognized the cost-savings rationale for central purchasing, but
they reported more drawbacks than advantages to them. For example, according to the director of dietary services, Norfield's
two units differed substantially in dietary costs because services
are not the same:

> There's a big difference between my department and
> the one at Bright. Other than the fact that our dietary
> supervisors are autonomous, I can't really tell you
> why. Bright, for example, uses disposable flatware.
> It's more expensive, but also the patients and em-
> ployees who eat in the cafeteria don't like it. An-
> other difference is that Bright serves steak ap-
> proximately twelve times every thirty days, whereas
> we serve steak maybe four times a month. . . .
> These differences don't sound like very much. How-
> ever, over a year's operations we spend over
> $100,000 less than Bright.

Some managers objected to the cost-savings claims on the
grounds that the costs of storage, paper work, and delivery eat up

the savings. For example, the director of dietary services remained unconvinced that the alleged benefits really were obtained:

> The biggest change in the last few years is the one in
> the purchasing system . . . but as far as I'm con-
> cerned, it hasn't justified itself economically. I just
> can't see how Norfield, with all the machinery and
> people involved in the extra handling, can save any
> money with this central purchasing theory. The
> original idea was to get other hospitals interested in
> the concept. However, this hasn't happened yet. I
> don't have any data, but I can't rationalize in my mind
> the equipment, the handling staff, and the storage ex-
> pense as being offset by the savings they claim. Out
> of my total monthly budget I would say that 20 percent
> of my purchases come from central supply. That ac-
> counts for about 75 percent of my headaches. One of
> the main problems is that we have no way of knowing
> if an item is available in supply until we order it.
> Another one is that whoever does the purchasing is
> often not aware of differences in quality so they are
> actually not saving money at all. They are buying
> lower priced but lower quality goods . . . they don't
> handle many perishables. Sometimes I find that I
> can better the price that central supply is paying.
> Their lack of uniformity and standardization in or-
> dering can actually cost the hospital money. . . .
> Sometimes I feel like whoever is doing our purchas-
> ing doesn't really know what they are buying.

Clearly, the change to centralized purchasing did not live up to its promise in the view of managers at the department-head level within Victory. The managers ascribed this situation to a combination of factors, such as rising prices, shifting away from name brands, and failure to set standards of quality across the member units of Norfield. They felt that coordination was inadequate, leading to a loss of confidence in the prescribed system.

DECENTRALIZATION AND DELEGATION

Despite the centralizing tendencies reflected in computerization and central purchasing, the idea of decentralization had a strong attraction for Victory's managers. Centralizing phenomena were tolerated as necessary for growth or cost-cutting, but individual managers took pride in delegating substantial authority and responsibilities to subordinates; subordinates admired and respected bosses who delegated effectively. Decentralization was real and not merely verbalized. Many managers thought that decentralization should be increased, and that delegation was the principal means to this end.

Decentralization as a policy was clearly apparent in the domain of the vice president for business administration. One of the financial counselors in Nelling's office described her as a good organizer and a good delegator, although he thought decentralization should be even greater:

> When I first came here it seemed as though no one was responsible for anything, and that everyone did any kind of work. That is, there was no real order around here. Therefore, it was decided that we needed to decentralize a lot of the duties in the business office and assign specific responsibilities. People in the office liked the idea and it was well accepted. However, I don't believe that this decentralization has gone as far as it should.

Growth is a kind of organizational change that fosters delegation, markedly changing the tasks and roles of managers. Work becomes more managerial in nature, as indicated by the director of dietary services:

> The main difference that I have experienced in this department over the years is that we've gone from a small unit to a large unit. The main effect of this change is that I'm not involved with patients any more and I have to delegate a lot of my responsibilities. My time seems to be taken up with interpreting organization policy, scheduling, and working out the problems of employees, such as holiday time and sick time.

Wright himself was proud of his ability to delegate. His subordinates perceived him to be an effective delegator, regarding him as an example worth following. In his view, all activities occurring in the hospital were his responsibility, but their magnitude made delegation an imperative:

> Interviewer: You have delegated quite a bit to your
>   vice presidents?

Wright: Yes, I have. Everything here is all my job,
it is just divided up among those who are here. I
have to exercise coordination and control but I
have to rely on all these other people to carry out
parts of the job. I'll give you an example. A
while back, we discovered that the income from
our parking deck was down and was going down
each month. Naturally, this was a concern. If
you'll look at the organizational chart, you will
see that under one vice president we have maintenance. They clean the deck. But the housekeeping department cleans the plaza. We also have a
Professional Office Building, which is the responsibility of Mrs. Nelling. What we discovered
is that everyone is partially involved, but no one
wanted to assume responsibility for the falling
parking lot revenue. I finally had to assign it
directly to someone.

Interviewer: How did you make the assignment?

Wright: A general rule in a case like this is to assign it to someone who really wants it. It's no
good to assign it to someone who is reluctant, so
I first have to look around to see who might like
to have the responsibility. I ask them to give me
their ideas. However, if nobody wants a function
like this, I don't hesitate to force it—I make the
assignment and it sticks.

Victory, like all hospitals, is a 24-hour-a-day, seven-days-
a-week operation. This delegation-producing fact was very much
in the awareness of all the managers interviewed. The chief administrator, the four vice presidents, and most department heads
worked in the daytime hours, five days a week. Hence a problem
is to delegate in such a way as to assure effective operations during
nights and weekends. These managers respected the delegation
process, and supported it by placing themselves on call at any time
they might be needed when absent. This was particularly true for
Wright, who occasionally worked on evenings or Saturdays.

The manner in which Wright used the delegation process to
foster innovation and change was apparent in his open system, in
formal approach to the assignment of departments to the two operating vice presidents. However, the vice presidents resisted
Wright's approach. Ellis explained why:

> Mr. Wright is used to having business administration
> types rather than hospital administration types
> around him. He likes to see that everybody gets
> rounded out, has a wide experience, so he assigns
> functions to us on that basis. You could never get
> him to organize professional areas all under one
> vice president and service areas under another. . . .
> Not long ago, he suggested that I switch jobs with
> Watson. He would take my group and I would take his
> group of departments. That would be absolutely terri-
> ble. I think his objective is to keep people alert, and
> learning new things. But it would sure change the
> chemistry of things and be very traumatic.

Other managers also strongly resisted Wright's delegation
process. For example, when the vice presidential level was
created, department heads formerly reporting to Wright were assigned to the vice presidents, in effect adding one level of organization. The chief radiological technician, for example, resisted
this change at first, but was eventually co-opted by Wright's persistence:

> I told Mr. Wright I didn't want to work for a vice
> president. I wanted to report directly to him. . . .
> Anyway, at one of our staff meetings he passed out
> a new organization chart and I could hardly wait to
> see where he had put me. I noticed my name under
> one of the vice presidents, but I saw an asterisk
> after it and I looked at the bottom of the page and it
> said "Will remain for the time being under the Ad-
> ministrator." After a while, however, the asterisk
> disappeared off the organization chart and I wound
> up where I am now.

The working relationship between Wright and the chief technician in radiology helped pave the way for the latter's ultimate acceptance of a new boss between himself and Wright:

> I always got along fine with Mr. Wright. I found that
> on most things I didn't have to go to him at all. He
> was a hard taskmaster, but I learned a lot from him.
> On a lot of things I didn't go to him because if I had
> all the facts, he wanted me to go ahead and make the
> decision myself. If I didn't have the facts, it was my
> job to get them . . . it wouldn't do any good to go to

him without a plan of action. I hated like hell for him
to give me to a vice president. But after working for
Mr. Wright, I figured I could take anybody. Don't
get me wrong when I say that. I don't mean anything
against Mr. Wright. I just mean that if you can work
for him, you can work for anyone else for sure.

Managerial change is facilitated by the respect, ability, and
strategies of a leader in whom subordinates have confidence. Con-
versely, the opposite is true also—innovation and change are
stymied to the extent that individuals lack confidence in their
leader. We can demonstrate this point further by examining the
department of nursing services at Victory.

DECENTRALIZATION AND DELEGATION
IN NURSING

The department of nursing services maintained a strong posture of decentralization through extensive delegation intended to
place subordinate units in positions of autonomy. Such a posture
would accord with the expectations of Wright, and would fit the
model of innovative, change-oriented management that was supposed
to prevail. These expectations, however, were more lip service
than actuality, as subordinate members of the nursing services
units saw them.

Nursing services, under the direction of Vice President Ella
Winters, was one of the largest units at Victory. Its staff of 650,
half that of the entire hospital, included 190 RNs, 180 LPNs, and a
number of nursing assistants, both male and female, plus unit
clerks for reception, intercoms, communication, and clinical
duties. (In some hospitals, unit clerks come directly under the
unit managers, but in Victory the unit clerks came under the nursing staff.)

Ella Winters had 15 unit coordinators reporting directly to
her. Each was in charge of one of the subdivisions, like emergency,
labor and delivery, the nursery, or intensive care units. Each of
these 15 was an RN. Winters was particular about their experience
and educational qualifications. In addition to the unit coordinators,
there were three assistant directors of nursing, one evening supervisor, and one night supervisor, all reporting to Winters.

These organizational relationships are shown in Figure 4.2,
which is drawn according to Winters's use of Likert's linking-pin
system. [6] Asked if she did not think this resulted in a rather wide
span of control, Winters replied that:

FIGURE 4.2

Linking-Pin Pattern of Nursing Services Organization in Victory Hospital

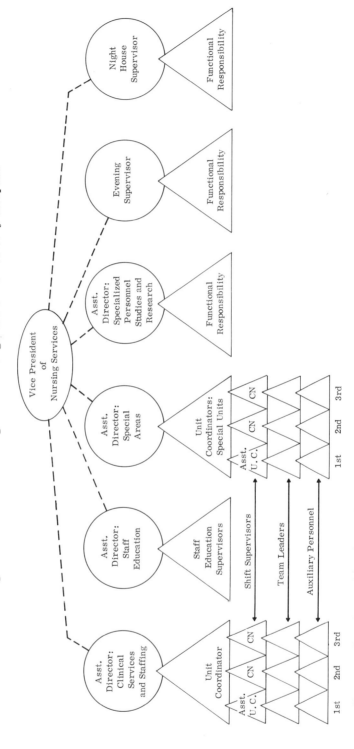

Source: Constructed by the author.

Well, I view our department as a decentralized system, with each of the unit coordinators taking full
responsibility on a 24-hour basis. If something goes
wrong at some point, the calls come to the unit coordinators. If somebody fails to show up on one of
the shifts, they have to get somebody or come in
themselves. I don't get calls about things like this.
We decentralize everything as much as possible,
including night and weekend duty.

Winters, though viewing her organization as "decentralized,"
stated that the 15 unit coordinators and the 3 assistant directors and
2 house supervisors, one for the evening shift and one for the night
shift, all reported directly to her. Her organization chart, however, shows the unit coordinators reporting to the assistant directors rather than directly to her. In a later interview, this discrepancy became better understood. Winters believed in delegation, and intended to delegate, but had reservations about the experience of the newly appointed assistant directors. Therefore,
although her span of control was technically five, she exercised
more direct authority over the unit coordinators than she preferred:

Most of the problems are routine and mundane and
should be delegated. However, I don't delegate some
of the work that I should because of the lack of ability
on the part of my assistant directors to accept responsibilities. Now I don't mean that they are not
adequate assistants. I mean that they haven't learned
the administrative skills necessary to accept some
types of responsibility. I believe the problem stems
from the fact that they see their roles differently from
the way I see them. That is, they go out to the units
every day and communicate and exchange ideas with
their unit coordinators and with their staff when they
should be staying in their office more and letting
these individuals make more decisions. They should
delegate more of their responsibilities and then I
would be able to delegate more of my responsibilities.
If the organization were decentralized to the extent
that I would like it, my assistant directors would be
shouldering more of the burden of the administrative
tasks such as coordinating, planning, linking, and
thinking. As it is now, they are very task oriented
and in effect are doing unit coordinator's jobs.

Despite problems of delegation, the nursing department at Victory was highly innovative and change-oriented. One innovation, for example, was the adoption of Likert's linking-pin organizational concept shown in Figure 4.2. According to this concept, the vice president, the four assistant directors, and the two house supervisors constitute a management group. Winters reflected this concept by stating that "There are few decisions which I am required to make alone." At the next level are the unit coordinators (nursing supervisors) and assistant directors with functional responsibilities such as staff education. These are viewed as links to the assistant unit coordinators who in turn direct the efforts of the nurses. Therefore they are pivotal to the whole concept. Another innovation was the team nursing system that is utilized instead of primary nursing care. This problem will be examined in detail in Chapter 6.

LEVELS OF INNOVATION

In this chapter, we have seen that organization structure and its associated management practices of delegating authority and responsibility provide a framework vital to the analysis of innovation and change. In particular, it is the degree of centralization or decentralization resulting from organization design and delegation that provides mechanisms for innovation and change processes. When coupled with the open-system attitudes characteristic of the top-level administrators, it becomes possible to foster and cope with demands for change arising at all levels.

There remains an important question as to the balance of administrative forces at work that produce innovation and change. At Victory, the levels of innovation and change corresponded closely to the levels of the organizational hierarchy. That is, the primary impetus was within the top echelons, the next most important level was the department heads, and the least important was in supervisory or technical areas. Moreover, the nature of the innovation or change necessarily shifts from broad, inclusive, major decisions to increasingly technical and operating types of decisions as one moves down the hierarchy. Wright reflected one reason for this:

> The top people can implement an innovation or suggestion or change at once. All I have to do is decide what I want. If I hear of a good idea, I can make the decision immediately. With innovations that arise further down in the organization, somebody has to sell the idea or persuade people to adopt it and this takes a lot more time and is sometimes discouraging to the innovator.

The research literature, particularly that devoted to participatory management and the open, adaptive organization, attaches great importance to lower hierarchical levels as sources of innovation and change. According to this view, there is a "bubbling up" of new ideas and practices arising out of the operating levels in touch with the scenes of daily action. However, there is also substantial evidence that top management levels are the most influential for innovation and change. The research on leadership points in this direction. Moreover, consultants and other practitioners insist on top management support in managing change.

Accordingly, a problem vital to understanding innovation and change is the fact that the sources of innovation and change do not fall in the same places in the hierarchy as do the sources of support or approval. Vigorous leadership can no doubt cause extensive, major change at critical turning points in the organization's history, but it is also the case that top leaders have the power to advance or block the efforts of change agents from below. This is why the degree of decentralization is an important factor. The greater the autonomy of units, the freer they are from administrative constraints on innovation and change.

Although it is clear that top management plays a strong role in innovation and change, Wright was generally unaware of the sources of contention between his own level and those further down. Wright was not only a strong advocate of innovation and change but was also in a powerful position for initiating, approving, or vetoing all but the most minor innovations and changes. His focus on the top level was expressed as follows:

> Well, I think innovation has to come from the top.
> There will be pockets of innovation that occur here
> and there in the organization and the administrator
> of course can support these pockets and draw them
> forth and encourage them. But I think the signifi-
> cant innovations come from the top. For example,
> I enjoy thinking about things and wondering what's
> new and keeping track of the possibilities for change
> and development. I find that keeping up with the
> daily routines aren't any fun. I could keep busy all
> the time listening to patient complaints and employee
> complaints, but that's not where the fun is. The fun
> comes from finding new and better ways to do some-
> thing we have been doing right along.

But when told that research findings support the critical importance of grass-roots innovation, Wright stated: "We need to know more about it." He suggested that perhaps different types of innovation occur at different levels.

Wilson has suggested that centralization is particularly important in the adoption phase of innovation because the top administrator must mediate contests between powerful subgroups. Conflicts make adoption and implementation a difficult process:

> . . . the adoption phase is a political activity and necessitates bargaining. When many high-power groups are engaged in the process, there is a strong tendency that there will be difficulty in reaching an accord, in which case adoption and implementation are not facilitated. [7]

TABLE 4.1

Differential Perceptions of Administrators, Medical
Department Heads, Physicians, and Trustees with
Respect to Adoption and Implementation
of Hospital-wide Changes

	Administrators	Staff
1. Administrative staff participation as viewed by administrative staff and administrator	Considerable	Considerable
2. Medical department heads participation as viewed by department heads and administration	Administrators / Considerable	Department heads / Some
3. Physician participation as viewed by physicians and administrator	Administrators / Considerable	Physicians / Some
4. Trustee participation as viewed by trustees and administrators	Administrators / Considerable	Trustees / Some

Source: Adapted from Arnold D. Kaluzny and James E. Veney, "Who Influences Decisions in the Hospital? Not Even the Administrator Really Knows," Modern Hospital, December 1972, pp. 52-53.

Kaluzny and Veney shed further light on the contending influences of power centers on adoption and implementation. They found that administrators claimed that department heads, physicians, and trustees have more influence on decisions than they perceive themselves as having. This suggests that participation has not been fully utilized as a managerial approach to greater organizational effectiveness. The discrepancy between reported involvement of various groups and the degree of involvement perceived by administrators could seriously impede efforts to involve them because the administrator perceives involvement as already existing. The adoption and implementation of hospital-wide changes was one of six decision areas examined in the Kaluzny and Veney study. Table 4.1 abstracts the summaries for this variable from the Kaluzny and Veney study.[8]

It is clear from the analysis thus far that the hospital administrator and his staff must do more than affirm the importance of innovation and change, and that their positive attitudes and postures are necessary but not sufficient conditions for innovation and change. Those interested in improving the management of innovation and change should review the impact of the degree of decentralization actually in effect, and further, should analyze the impacts of their relationship to the key subgroups within their organization.

A more detailed assessment of ideation, adoption, and implementation will be presented in the chapters to follow.

NOTES

1. Jon L. Pierce and Andre L. Delbecq, "Organization Structure, Individual Attitudes, and Innovation," Academy of Management Review 2 (January 1977): 30-31.

2. Ibid., p. 31.

3. James P. Cooney and Thomas L. Alexander, Part One, "Overview," in Multihospital Systems: An Evaluation (Evanston, Ill.: Health Services Research Center, Northwestern University, 1975), p. 1.

4. Victor A. Thompson, Bureaucracy and Innovation (University: University of Alabama Press, 1969), pp. 98-99.

5. Ibid.

6. Rensis Likert, New Patterns of Organization (New York: McGraw-Hill, 1961), pp. 113-15.

7. James Q. Wilson, "Innovation and Organization: Notes toward a Theory," in Approaches to Organization Design, ed. James D. Thompson (Pittsburgh: University of Pittsburgh Press, 1966), p. 392.

8. Arnold D. Kaluzny and James E. Veney, "Who Influences Decisions in the Hospital? Not Even the Administrator Really Knows," Modern Hospital, December 1972, pp. 52-53.

5

HUMAN CAPABILITIES

To continue our examination of the first stage of the model presented in Figure 1.3, we shall now examine the influences of human capabilities on innovation and change within the context of organization structure and management styles in Victory Hospital. We shall briefly consider the environmental context of the creative imagination. We will then analyze selected human capabilities: professionalism, morale and motivation, and the values of organization members. Finally, we will see how the personnel function had limited effects on innovation and change.

THE CREATIVE ENVIRONMENT

All who enter the main lobby of Victory Hospital encounter a tranquil physical space tastefully decorated in warm colors and equipped with new and comfortable furnishings. The area itself is spacious, though often crowded with waiting people and briskly moving members of the hospital staff. Just off the lobby is a passage to the main elevators and to offices and waiting rooms for laboratories and the admitting office. The walls of this passageway are covered with original works of art by local artists. The pictures, which are for sale, are changed each month so that one constantly encounters new manifestations of beauty. Throughout the building, in offices and hallways, tasteful reproductions and original paintings abound. The light and cheerful décor and the abundance of plants, artwork, and attractive furnishings produce an attractive working environment conducive to creativity.

The physical environment of the hospital is not, however, everywhere pleasant. Sickness and pain are pervasive, and employees may be depressed over constant contacts with suffering patients, distraught relatives, and the detritus resulting from efforts to help the sick. Maintenance and other workers inhabit subterranean locations where they work on grubby machinery and noisy equipment. Congestion and confusion abound where employees and other people come together in large numbers, such as cafeterias or waiting rooms. It is plainly difficult to eliminate from the physical or human environments much that depresses or stultifies.

Even more important and more subtle is the presence of organization structure together with administrative styles and philosophies and the resulting sociopsychological climate. Organization climates reflect the feelings and attitudes of the members. This climate results from many forces, including technology, structure, and the behavior of the members themselves and their managers. The research literature suggests that task environments, such as objectives, procedures, and controls, and organization structures both stimulate and inhibit the creativity of individuals. But the evidence is inconclusive concerning which variables tend to facilitate or dampen creativity, and how their influence actually works.

In an experimental study, Cummings, Hinton, and Gobdel conclude that the attributes of a task environment, either individually or collectively, have strong, consistent effects on creative performance. However, they found that explicit objectives (instructions) to be creative increase creative performance and that control and monitoring procedures inhibit it. Introducing specific procedures on how to be creative had no significant impact. Since the effects of structure and task environment on creativity vary across several dimensions, and across specific measures of creativity, they recommend caution about general statements concerning the pervasive impact of task environment or structural variables on creative performance.[1]

Similarly, Maddi has expressed skepticism about situational views of creativity: "What I am skeptical about is that the persons who need such a felicitous environment would ever be able to manage creativity in the real world of varying and uncontrollable environments." He doubts that attempts to spur creativity by unstructured and permissive environments can have more than temporary effects. Considering the nature of human beings, he believes that the impetus for creativity must be very frail if it can be significantly curtailed by structured, evaluative environments.[2]

Victory, with its paradoxical bureaucratic structure, coupled with the open-system attitudes of the top administrators, achieved a working balance between the views of those who emphasize structural variables and those who advocate open systems as the means of generating creativity. To appraise Victory's capabilities for creative change, Corwin's study proved useful. In a survey of sociological research on organizational change, Corwin lists seven postulates drawn from existing diverse and overlapping streams of research. These are presented in Table 5.1, along with a broad assessment of the extent to which they apply to Victory Hospital. It can be seen in this table that the first four postulates pertain to the characteristics of people, while the last three denote organizational characteristics.[3] In general, Victory Hospital achieves a high standing on two of the human capability postulates and three of the organizational context postulates.

INFLUENCES ON CREATIVITY

Creativity as the product of individual effort has been extensively analyzed, but mainly through subjective commentary or the introspections of creative persons, such as actors, writers, or composers.[4] In general, however, innovators are more likely to be organizational employees than individuals acting alone, and more likely to be highly educated, as in the case of scientists and engineers. People do not create in a vacuum. Rather they rise to meet challenges through active search for solutions to problems. Novel solutions are more likely to be accepted if they fit the overall strategies, preferences, and decision techniques of an organization.[5]

Knight has summarized the conclusions of existing research about the creative problem-solving process. Table 5.2 lists six characteristics of creative people, along with an assessment of how the findings at Victory relate to them.[6] Victory's employees appeared to be high in devotion to work, receptivity, exploration and search, and low in risk acceptance and nonconformity.

The chaplain, who reported directly to the chief administrator, occupied a strategic position for observing creativity. He had broad responsibilities for pastoral care and the counseling of patients and their families. He also directed a clinical training program, consisting of ministerial interns and participants in a one-year postgraduate program and a three-month summer program. Since his functions kept him close to the hospital's main components, and he reported directly to Wright, he was familiar with an array of human problems throughout the organization. Moreover, his training (eight years for certification as one of five clinical training supervisors in the United States) gave him special capabilities for observation. His starting point was the role of creativity in theology: creativity as ongoing creation, a fundamental tenet in most religions.

TABLE 5.1

Applicability of Postulates on Organization Change
in Victory Hospital

	Applicability to Victory Hospital	
Postulates	High	Medium

An organization can be more readily
changed if:

		High	Medium
1.	It is invaded by liberal, creative, and unconventional outsiders with fresh perspectives.	X	
2.	Those outsiders are exposed to creative, competent socialization agents.		X
3.	It is staffed by young, flexible socialization agents.		X
4.	Its members have positions that are sufficiently secure and protected from the status risks involved in change.	X	
5.	It is structurally complex and decentralized.	X	
6.	It has the outside funds to provide the organizational slack necessary to lessen the cost of innovation.	X	
7.	It is located in a changing, modern, urbanized setting where it is in close cooperation with a coalition of other cosmopolitan organizations that can supplement its skills and resources.	X	

Source: Adapted from Ronald G. Corwin, "Strategies for Organizational Innovation," American Sociological Review 37 (August 1972): 441-54.

TABLE 5.2

Characteristics of Creative People in Victory Hospital

Characteristic	Applicability to Victory Hospital		
	High	Medium	Low
1. Creative problem solving appears to be a high-risk activity, that is, often erratic and unpredictable.			X
2. Creative people appear to have a detached devotion to their work; they have a deep commitment to the problem they are trying to solve, yet they are not so deeply immersed that they are unable to see the problem in a broader perspective.	X		
3. Creative people are receptive to all kinds of ideas. They will consider them and judge them on their merits.	X		
4. Creative people rely on free exploration in that they actively go out and search for new alternatives, advice, ideas, and opinions from a wide variety of sources.	X		
5. Creative individuals appear to commit themselves to specific solutions to their problems later than their less creative counterparts.		X	
6. Creative people tend to be nonconformists and question authority and existing problem solutions.			X

Source: Adapted from Kenneth E. Knight, "A Descriptive Model of the Intra-firm Innovation Process," Journal of Business 40, no. 4 (October 1967): 481.

The chaplain did not believe that Victory was achieving its potential for creative approaches to hospital problems. He also saw people as the primary source of momentum for improvement and change.

> Interviewer: Your work seems to be well within the sector of creativity.
> Chaplain: Yes, it is. However, we are not up to our potential in this area. We don't do all we could to be innovative and creative.
> Interviewer: What do you think makes an organization creative?
> Chaplain: The main thing is to be open to change. We've got to try not to be rigid with personalities. People are all different. They mustn't be threatened by an idea that is not accepted in theory.
> Interviewer: That's very interesting.
> Chaplain: You can't wait around for permission from the top. The top has to be open, to allow feedback, and let innovation rise to the top.
> Interviewer: That's something of a paradox, isn't it? Some feel that leaders provide the innovation and creativity and others say the leaders don't know anything operational so it has to come from the bottom.
> Chaplain: Well, I think Mr. Manton and Mr. Wright are both idea-producing people. They are turned on by ideas. They perceive their task in large part as fostering innovation and creativity and it takes a lot of ability to allow sufficient freedom. My job is to interpret our activities to them so that they can make intelligent allocations of resources and maintain the flow of innovation.

The chaplain emphasized trust among people and the acceptance of risk as important factors fostering creativity and innovation. The informants in this study perceived varying degrees of trust in the organization. The chaplain felt that trust was low in some departments, among them nursing, and high in others.

> Chaplain: Another big element is trust.
> Interviewer: Is trust widespread in this organization?
> Chaplain: No, it isn't. The level of trust is very low in some departments but trust is facilitated in other departments. You have to work at developing

trust. You have to allow for positive and negative
feedback. You have to deal aggressively as well
as defensively with ideas. Also, you have to take
risks. To permit people to take the risks that innovation entails, one must have trust. Some of
this trust is in the individual. An individual needs
to have a great deal of trust. If a person is self-
confident and secure, he can take more risks.

Interviewer: The idea of risk is very interesting.

Chaplain: People evaluate the risk factor when they
check out new ideas. We've got the past history
of our lives to go by. People project probabilities and "hunch out" the system. They are not always aware they are doing these things, but they
do it.

Interviewer: They send up trial balloons?

Chaplain: That's right. They are always planting
seeds or putting up trial balloons.

Asked for an example of lack of trust, the chaplain observed
that he saw this as a problem in the nursing department:

Chaplain: The nursing coordinators feel that they
have no part in effective change. Change is from
the top down. Now this isn't any one person's fault.
It's something like in a religious order. It's hard
to get participation and to get the negative feedback
that is needed. Some people feel that ideas should
be shelved. There's a lot of indifference in the
organization but at least resisters have taken account of negative feedback and we need that. Some
people feel threatened and others don't.

Interviewer: It's much like that in all types of organizations, isn't it?

Chaplain: Yes, it is. It's almost like the parent-
child relationship the way we behave in organizations.

The director of nursing supported the chaplain's views about
the level of trust at Victory, although not in her own department:

Interviewer: Do you have a lot of trust at Victory?

Winters: No, I'm not so sure that I can say that
we do. Everything is uphill all the way. It's
pretty easy for us to be complacent or over-

confident. I don't think the element of trust in
each other is what it ought to be.

Winters also expressed strong feelings about the role of creativity
as a skill needed to free nurses from the bonds of tradition:

Creativity should be a basic skill because most nurses
maintain tradition and have a tendency to question
change. Commonly, the attitude is that something
has always worked one way, so why change it? Routine approaches to patient care have a way of ration-
alizing problems and overlooking better ways of
helping patients. I feel that creativity will give a
nursing supervisor some general flexibility to face
these traditional problems of nursing and maybe
reduce such things as patient complaints.

Argyris has asserted that innovative activity can be expected
to be greater when top management abandons "pyramidal values,"
recruits creative, competent people, and develops a high-trust atmosphere. Also, he found that innovativeness is higher in young
organizations than in old ones, and that after a honeymoon period
in the growth of a young organization, innovation may become stifled
by complex structure, the incompetence of people, and increasingly
tight controls.[7] At Victory, hierarchical (pyramidal) values received less emphasis than in many bureaucracies. High-competence
people occupied medical, technical, middle-management, and top
management positions. Victory was also relatively young as an
organization in its present form. On the other hand, there were
pockets of low trust and a high level of administrative control
through records, reports, cost-benefit analysis, and supervisory
monitoring.

It can be concluded that both the personal attributes of people
and organizational context variables interact to influence the creativity of members in complex ways. We will now take a closer look at
the human capabilities of individuals at work in Victory Hospital.

PROFESSIONALS AND INNOVATION

Hospital organizations encompass an array of professional,
semiprofessional, and technical personnel who espouse values of
autonomy and independence. Their occupational outlooks tend to
set them apart from ordinary employees and their ties with outside
associations provide them with a community of discourse that
reaches beyond the hospital.

Summarizing a large number of studies, Pierce and Delbecq develop the proposition that "professionalism will be positively related to organizational innovation." They found strong agreement that professionalism brings to an organization a richness of experience, self-confidence, ideation from outside sources, increased boundary spanning, professional standards, and psychological commitment to moving beyond the status quo. These conditions are viewed as conducive to the innovative process. [8]

Cosmopolitan attitudes and behavior (orientations to outside loyalties and directives) are characteristic of professionals. Cosmopolitanism has been found to be positively associated with program innovation, [9] and the cosmopolitan orientation of administrators and organizational staff was found by Kaluzny, Veney, and Gentry to be a predictor of innovation in health care organizations. [10]

The research at Victory supports the Pierce and Delbecq proposition and the findings of other researchers on the influence of professionalization. We have already shown that professional activities and attitudes contribute to ideation through boundary spanning, enriched experience, and commitment to change. The short tenures and readiness to change jobs found among top administrators at Victory and Norfield further illustrate the mobility and cosmopolitan characteristics of professionals.

There is, however, another view that research has not yet thoroughly explained: professionalism has its awkward moments, its limitations. Moreover, the existence of professionals, including managers who hold professional attitudes, poses difficult problems of administration. The connections between professionals and innovative processes are mediated by problems of control, coordination, integration, and utilization, and their associated frustrations.

CONTROL

At Victory, the loose control of personnel was seen to be a widespread problem. According to the assistant director of nursing, for example, disciplinary actions were difficult to take among professionals such as registered nurses:

> Interviewer: Are any sanctions imposed on RNs or
>   staff nurses who don't conform to the guidelines
>   laid down by Mrs. Winters or by the specialized
>   personnel ?
> Assistant Director: Hardly ever. Unit coordinators
>   are hesitant to "conference" registered nurses.
>   A conference is where a person is written up for

not doing his assigned task in the assigned manner.
I don't necessarily agree with this practice. As a
matter of fact, I feel that RNs are professionals.
I don't like to see professionals not be professional
and fail to accept their responsibilities. I believe
Mrs. Winters is beginning to change her attitudes
in this respect. Until recently a unit coordinator
was not mandated to do anything. Mrs. Winters
believes in creative leadership and so do I, but
she felt that unit coordinators were taking advantage of her. For example, she had suggested that
they get to know every subordinate by changing
shifts and that they get to work early in the morning before the shift changes. But some of them
won't do it.

Winters also felt that her assistant directors were not sufficiently professional. They were too heavily engaged in technical
work which inhibited their creativity and innovation:

I haven't quite gotten them there yet and I still do a lot
of routine, mundane tasks because of their inability.
I feel that a nursing supervisor, regardless of what
level she's on, should be able to plan, think, create,
and implement. These four basic functions I feel are
very important, and we're not doing enough of these
things.

As in other organizations, control was a pervasive force in
Victory Hospital. Bureaucratic control procedures represent a
type of influence likely to inhibit innovation and change because they
reduce the autonomy of managers and constrain those who are controlled. In Victory, control pressure was heavy at department head
and supervisory levels, though lighter at the top where the administrator, the vice presidents, and the chaplain professed open organization views.
Controls at the department head and supervisory levels emphasized task performance, conformity to rules, evaluation procedures, records, costs, and budgets. The functioning of these
control mechanisms left little scope for the encouragement of managerial innovation and change, although technical or procedural innovations occurred frequently at these levels. In the nursing group,
for example, "conferencing" emphasized control and discipline
rather than its developmental possibilities. According to a unit
coordinator:

One of my primary duties is the annual evaluation of the nursing staff. It's a time-consuming ordeal for me. Part of the evaluation process is a conference with each nurse prior to making an evaluation. For instance, if someone is not doing the job or maintaining the quality standards we insist on, I conduct a conference with that employee and tell her what I have observed and ask her what the problem is. Then we'll try to find a solution. This is a better and fairer way to do the evaluations. What I mean by fair is that human errors, such as in medication, will happen. Therefore, we want to get all the facts before we make an evaluation. These conferences are recorded and signed by the individuals and they go into the file. Of course, a conference can be for something good as well as bad.

Control processes included several types of sanctions, depending on the departmental policy. For example, reprimands through "counseling" or "conferencing" were found in environmental services and nursing. According to the director of environmental services:

Director: I've had 57 counselings or reprimands since the first of January 1974. I consider this rather heavy. Greater than any place I've ever worked before.

Interviewer: Can you tell me more about these counselings?

Director: A counseling is an official reprimand that becomes part of an employee's permanent record. For example, if a supervisor sees that an employee shows up late for work or doesn't do what he's supposed to or leaves work early or generally gets out of line, he'll send me an informal note about it. I then type up a counseling form that becomes part of the permanent record of the employee. I'm stricter than most of the directors of the departments in the hospital and I keep these personnel evaluations very accurately. Therefore, when I fire a person, he stays fired. I try to be fair with my employees and not use these evaluations as a weapon. However, I also want my employees to know what's expected of them and to do it. . . .

Incident reports, similar to "conferences," were used to control troubles that might cause the hospital litigation. The assistant director of special studies in nursing had the responsibility for screening all incident reports, which are written up by the staff whenever an incident occurs that concerns either patients, employees, or visitors. The primary purpose is to consider possible litigation.

In more technical areas also the managers expressed strong needs for autonomy based on professional attributes as well as personnel preferences. Yet the limitations of control were clearly apparent. For example, the manager of the business office reported that he had "autonomy" over spending money on training programs, but "I'm very task-oriented in that I believe in getting the job done. Mrs. Nelling seems happy as long as I do just that, get the job done. Of course, I know there are limitations to my job and I don't do anything I feel I shouldn't without getting her approval."

Similarly, in the department of inhalation therapy, the director indicated frustrations over the conflict between autonomy and control:

> When I went to work here eight years ago, Mr. Wright
> said he wanted me to run the department as I saw fit.
> I believe I've held up my end of the bargain and the
> situation has worked well. Now I'm not saying that it's
> all been peaches and cream, because all of my ideas
> haven't been accepted. For instance, my requests for
> bigger raises for my subordinates have almost always
> been turned down.

MORALE, MOTIVATION, AND VALUES

According to Pierce and Delbecq, the attitudinal, motivational, and value states of an organization's members play a critical role in predicting innovation. Their survey of the research literature shows that (1) some models of innovation are based on motivational concepts, (2) innovative behavior depends on whether organization members view themselves as successful or unsuccessful, (3) job dissatisfaction is positively associated with the rate of program change, (4) satisfied members search for ways to improve conditions and to be more receptive to new ideas, (5) internal commitments and a sense of intrinsic rewards lead to the initiation of innovative ideas, and (6) a strong identification with one's work may be a viable predictor of innovation.[11]

The findings at Victory lend strong support to four propositions derived by Pierce and Delbecq: (1) job satisfaction and job
involvement will be positively related to innovation, (2) performance
dissatisfaction will be positively related to innovation, (3) intrinsic
motivation will be positively related to motivation, and (4) values of
strategic decision makers favorable toward change will be positively
related to organizational innovation.

We have already shown that at Victory innovation was perceived as being relatively high, and that the values of strategic decision makers were favorable toward change. We can now look more
closely at attitudes toward work, jobs, and people in order to observe their impact on innovation.

Levels of morale and motivation among the managers and employees at Victory Hospital were generally high. This was evident
at all levels and across the various departments. For example, in
admitting, the director indicated a sense of importance of the admitting function which influenced his ability to bring about change:

> Interviewer: I gather the idea for streamlining the de-
> partment was yours. Is that right?
> Director: Yes, that was my idea. The reason I felt
> that it was necessary to implement this change
> was simply because I hate lost motion. I believe
> the idea was a natural result of my attitude about
> admitting. I feel that most people don't under-
> stand how important admitting is in the hos-
> pital. . . . It takes a very cool, calm individual
> to handle the various situations that can arise here.

Although no formal suggestion system was in use at Victory,
upward communication was invited in an effort to improve morale
through a call-line system for combating rumors and answering
questions:

> Ellis: We just finished instituting a new idea called
> the "call line." It's for employees or administra-
> tors. They can dial a phone number and give their
> comments or questions, and we promise that they
> will get a response. They can gripe or bitch, say
> whatever they want to. We've gotten about 150
> calls to date.
> Interviewer: How do you respond?
> Ellis: Sometimes we write them an answer to give
> them information or we may talk to them directly.
> We do get some weird inputs. Most of the things

are innocuous, like when are we going to get a
salary increase or my fenders got smashed in
the parking lot. Some of the things we can't do
much about.

A similar avenue for upward communication was found in the
department of environmental services. It, too, was useful in administering the processes of change. A periodic "gripe session"
was held, according to the director:

Interviewer: Do you feel that these gripe sessions
are beneficial? Do they help?
Director: A lot of things come out. Sometimes
there's name calling and sometimes there's useful criticism. For example, I found out that the
employees resented a new assistant I hired. The
reason I had gotten the new assistant was that we
needed to get some order back into our cleaning
procedures and I thought that she could rewrite
some of the procedures. Obviously, the employees saw her as a threat to their jobs. Problems like this are not unique here.

That morale was generally high at Victory was in no small
measure due to attitudes of confidence in subordinates. It was reflected in a feeling of congeniality among working associates. Commitment, loyalty, and cohesiveness were frequently alluded to at
all levels, but the higher levels set the pattern. For example,
Ellis, who supervised nine operating department heads, stated that:

We've had a very stable group, and a good group.
They feel good about their work and feel good about
being with us. They all have substantial longevity.
I am confident in them and I know I can count on
them. . . . If you look at the resumes of these department heads, they might seem kind of ordinary
but they are a unique kind of people. I have to
credit Mr. Wright with building the kind of organization here that has one extra ingredient--idealism,
the belief in what we're doing and commitment on
the part of most people.

Similarly, the physician in charge of the pathology laboratory
reported that:

> I think we've got the best people in any hospital any-
> where around. If I sound charged up over this, it's
> because I really do feel that way. I think we've got
> the best medical staff of any hospital in the world.
> We've got people who will take on anything you ask
> them to. They will take on big jobs. All we have
> to do is ask them.

The assistant director for staff education in the nursing department, a relatively new position, reported similarly that:

> As President Ford might say, "My group is still in
> the honeymoom phase." They are exceptional people
> and simply because of the fact that we respect each
> other, we manage to work in harmony with one an-
> other. I'm really not sure why we get along so well
> together. It may have something to do with the fact
> that we know each other very well. . . . All I can
> really say is that we appreciate and respect one
> another and I feel that's very important.

Congeniality was highlighted by several informants as a characteristic of their work group. The chief pharmacist, for example,
said that "the atmosphere in the pharmacy is congenial. Everyone
works well together." And the director of medical records indicated that ". . . I believe the fact that the people in this hospital
work so well together is one reason I have been working here for
29 years. This attitude of congeniality I believe is reflected from
the top of the organization down."

Fairness of a supervisor appears to be an important consideration with respect to job attitudes. According to one of the typists
in the admitting department:

> The director is a very fair person and I like her
> very much. As a matter of fact, she's so fair that
> she's almost unfair. I mean, she really leans over
> backwards and goes out of her way to help someone
> or to tolerate an employee until he can straighten
> himself out.

The primary factors inhibiting high morale and motivation
were pay problems and the demands for conformity coupled with
close supervision. For example, a hospital policy allowing pay
differentials for those gaining certification in their specialties was
abolished. Also, the night-shift differential for inhalation therapists

was removed, although, as the therapists were well aware, night-shift differentials existed for other occupations, such as nursing. According to the director, a wage and salary study by outside consultants actually lowered the wage rates in his department and led to lower morale.

How innovation and change are related to supervisory attitudes toward subordinates is illustrated in the adoption of a new biomedical equipment maintenance program. The consultant who assisted in the development of this program was also retained as a part-time employee to instruct workers in the new system:

> Interviewer: So the point of your instruction is not just to familiarize new technicians with the equipment but also to give them an appreciation of what is going on in the entire hospital?
>
> Consultant: That's it exactly. We had a man not long ago that felt that women on the nursing wards were the most ornery things he had ever seen. I could see a bad situation developing, so I got him to start making daily rounds on these floors and asking these women how their work was going and checking equipment. He soon got to like most of the people and was talking to them. His attitude seemed to change 100 percent. One of the reasons I became involved in this biomedical maintenance program is that I got interested in these people and what they are trying to do.

The biomedical maintenance consultant also gave respect a higher priority than money as an influence on motivation and morale:

> If administration could spend a little more time seeing what goes into maintaining all this equipment, I believe they would appreciate maintenance a little more than they do and would show a little more respect. What these people need just as much as money is respect. For what they are paid, they do a damn good job. . . . The men at the top of the organization in ivory towers don't have any idea what their employees' problems are. I feel that the way things are changing and the new problems that are developing, better communication and appreciation is a good safety valve.

In the lower levels of the organization, many of the department heads and supervisors resisted the employees' need for autonomy, insisting on close supervision and conformity to rules and standards. These attitudes posed a striking contrast to their postures of congeniality and having confidence in people as morale builders. The following are illustrative comments from three informants:

> I have to keep my eyes on the employees to make sure they don't start playing doctor or getting careless and overstepping the bounds of their responsibility.

> You have to check practically everything that these types of people do. . . . People on the low end of the pay scale are, generally speaking, not well motivated and you have to keep tabs on them.

> The one big problem I encounter is getting employees to conform—to do what they are told to do, to get to work on time, to be where they are supposed to be, to do the job that they are assigned. I personally believe that the underlying motive for their resistance is that they just don't like directions. They dislike taking orders. They want to go and come at their own pleasure.

Motivational principles were basic to one of the most successful innovations at Victory: the development of a new incentive system for the typists in the typing pool for medical record transcription. The plan called for paying them on an incentive basis beyond 500 lines of transcribing a day.

The idea for the medical record transcribers incentive system came from Wright. He and Ben Watson jointly implemented the new idea. The director of medical services indicated that the group's output averaged three times the national average of words per day. Under the new system, turnover was generally lower and group morale was higher. Significantly, the implementation of this basic idea was followed shortly thereafter by the initiation and implementation of a derivative idea by the typists. According to Wright:

> . . . On their own, the typists came up with the idea that while the automatic typing machines were retyping the corrected data from tapes, [drafts are made first and the corrected copies automatically printed out] they could be typing on another machine. So they asked for an additional machine and while one

machine is running they are typing on the other.
This boosts their earnings and their output.

Clearly, high motivation and morale at Victory led to group
cohesion, a sense of fairness, and higher performance. Deliberately cultivated, these characteristics appear to lead to ideation and
spur adoption and implementation. We shall now examine the management of the personnel function in the light of its contribution to
innovation and change.

SELECTION PROCEDURES

The effort to assess potential for creativity and innovation in
prospective employees at Victory was minimal, although the ability
and motivation to learn were highly valued. The primary sources
for recruiting candidates were professional or technical schools,
word-of-mouth dissemination of vacancy information by current
employees, and the appearance of candidates at the personnel office
to inquire about openings.

Scarcities of supply in a number of key fields, coupled with
reliance on interviews conducted by supervisory personnel or department heads following the filling out of an application blank, led
to the hiring of employees more on the basis of expediency than on
sophisticated systematic screening processes designed to discover
capabilities beyond the merely technical.

Nursing, a high turnover group, illustrates the difficulty of
assessing the potential for creativity and innovation through the
methods used at Victory. One of the assistant directors of nursing,
asked if the ability to innovate could be assessed in selection interviews, stated that:

Assistant Director: Sometimes it's possible. It's
hard to be sure what information you are getting
from the early interviews with a candidate. A
lot of them will just go along with what you are
driving at in order to get the job. I don't believe
we can really judge this factor very much in applicants. A lot of them really do not talk much.
Interviewer: Would you like to be able to make a
better estimate of this factor if you could?
Assistant Director: Yes, I think so. I like applicants who ask a lot of questions. Then I feel
that they are interested and that they would be
an asset to the hospital.

Interviewer: Do the applicants sometimes make
suggestions?

Assistant Director: Not too often. Most of them are
hesitant. However, they are from outside and
they've worked in other places. They do have
good ideas. We have a high turnover, so the fact
that we are getting a lot of new people all the time
helps bring in new ideas. A lot of them we can't
use, but it is one source.

The idea of getting innovation through "new blood" stemming
from high turnover was echoed by Watson, though he was doubtful
that significant innovation could be obtained this way:

In selecting people for positions or in assigning
duties, I can't really tie that in with innovation too
much. Of course, when somebody new comes in,
you always get new blood but may or may not get
useful innovation and I don't see any way to look for
it or to predict where it's going to exist. Like I
said, I've been here two years and I'm still learning.
It's sort of a trial and error system, a never ending
process. I would hope that my people would feel the
same way.

Vice President Ellis, however, felt differently:

I haven't had to recruit a department head yet.
That's where it would be a problem. I believe innovation should be a strong criterion in selecting
and rewarding people. A lot of people are very
competent, but they are not innovators. We don't
have big structures below the department head
levels so innovation is important among the department heads. However, I also want to be sure
of their operating skills.

Despite the absence of innovation criteria in the selection and
reward systems there was a definite belief throughout Victory that
innovation comes from innovative, aggressive individuals. But beneath this widespread acceptance were feelings about the need for
controls and restraints on ideation. For example, Vice President
Watson accepted the hiring of mavericks, but wanted them kept
under control.

Interviewer: Should you hire people for their ability
    to innovate?

Watson: A lot of this problem with innovation is up
    to the individual, so if you found an aggressive
    guy, he might dump a lot of ideas into the hopper.

Interviewer: Should you occasionally hire an oddball
    or misfit, so that you might get some unusual
    ideas?

Watson: Yes, if he is loyal and you can keep him
    under control. I would do it by holding him re-
    sponsible and holding my department heads re-
    sponsible. If the guy is way out in left field you
    have to hold him back. So a lot depends on me.

The same pattern—ideation under control—was present also
in the thinking of Vice President Nelling:

Interviewer: Do you have idea people who do nothing
    but come up with new ideas?

Nelling: No, we don't need people just sitting around.
    We want everybody to be doing something produc-
    tive. You have to be involved in what's going on.
    You can't use textbook approaches to solve prob-
    lems. You don't get any answers that way. There
    are so many factors that affect a problem that what
    is ideal for one organization like Victory might not
    be ideal at Bright. We make as wide a use of
    every idea as we can in our system but it is often
    hard to. An idea doesn't always cut across the
    whole setup.

Interviewer: What about people with wild, original
    ideas? What would happen to them?

Nelling: I think they would get a hearing. We need
    to solve problems around here, and no matter how
    crazy the individual is I think the idea itself would
    be evaluated on its merits.

Interviewer: Some writers have said that most
    creative and innovative people are mavericks,
    and not very likable people.

Nelling: That depends a lot on who does the hiring
    and the kind of personnel policies you have and
    what kind of people you get. As I've said, we
    can't just get people to sit around and think up
    ideas. They have to do some work and take part
    in the activities that are important around here.

>But anyone can get a hearing for his idea around
>here no matter how odd he is.

The fact that Victory is relatively innovative without trying to select creative people produces a paradox: in the absence of a formal personnel management function concentrating on innovation and creativity, some source other than employee selection must account for the high level of innovation and change. Many changes, as shown earlier, are forced by external events or internal necessities of various kinds, but even these as well as innovative changes appear to be highly localized and highly specific to a unit rather than the result of an organizational system specifically intended to produce creativity, innovation, and planned change. Most of the supervisors interviewed reported examples of their approach to getting more and better work out of their subordinates. A strong sense of mission and purpose, coupled with turnover and growth, makes a certain amount of innovation and change occur even without the influence of staff specialists such as personnel managers. For example, this occurred in the cardiovascular laboratory:

>Interviewer: Whose idea was it to create the job of
>cardiovascular technician?
>Laboratory Director: It was my idea. When I first
>came to Victory there was a 60-year-old ward
>clerk and a nurse running the catheterization lab.
>However, after a while we moved these people out
>and moved some good people in who had the skills
>to do the jobs that were necessary. We're every-
>where in the hospital, or we try to be, without
>anyone knowing we're there. All that's important
>is that the MD knows we are there and has confi-
>dence in what we are doing.

And in the department of environmental service, the director said, "Since I've been here we've tried to involve the employees more in the planning function and in revising procedure."

The selection process at Victory is not the kind that would be likely to result in the hiring of a large number of unusually creative people. Occasionally, however, a maverick slips through. Among those interviewed at all levels, perhaps no more than five could be labeled mavericks—persons who care more about change, improvement, or innovation than about their own reputations as "good guy," "cooperator," or "friendly, easy-going person." Ellis indicated that one of his department heads was such a person: "Casey is one of our bright young man types. He's an administrative nightmare to some people around here because of his energy and ambition. . . ."

Watson, the other operations vice president, appeared to be tolerant of idea-producing people:

Interviewer: Oddballs are hard to have around. They don't fit in, do they?

Watson: Well, that's alright. I think everybody should get a hearing. We should at least talk to people when they have something on their mind. If they can justify and support their thinking, then it's O.K.

Although the Victory organization did not succeed in hiring as many creative people as he thought it should, the hospital's chaplain felt that the selection process could make a good contribution toward this objective:

Interviewer: Can innovation be improved by selecting the right kind of people in an organization?

Chaplain: Yes, I think so. We can hire creative, secure people who have known track records of success. There is a famous football coach who will take on his team from high school only those who have been on winning teams. He doesn't want anybody who has had the experience of losing. So he gets all the people who know only success.

Watson felt that utilization of people was more of a problem than selection:

Interviewer: What groups at Victory are most in need of innovation?

Watson: Well, nursing, for one. There is more going into this all the time. There are a lot of changes in nursing which we ought to consider. Also, I think laboratories, especially the problem of better utilization of personnel. Also, I think we need more changes and improvements in admitting.

Interviewer: In labs, is it a problem of selection or something like that?

Watson: Not really selection, but a misutilization of people. You don't need a lab technician to spend time carrying trays across the street, for example. We've got to match the work to the level of training involved.

In several instances, chiefly technological in character, particular people were hired for the specific purpose of making innovative changes. For example, the manager of food services was hired upon his retirement from the army, and he brought outside expertise to Victory in the form of operating changes:

> Interviewer: Can you think of any innovation that you
> have been involved in in the time that you have
> worked at Victory?
> Manager: Most of the innovations or changes that I
> have been involved in are in our operating systems.
> An example is the food control system that I helped
> set up in the stock room. . . . Setting up new op-
> erating systems and maintaining them was some-
> thing I had been doing in the army for years. As a
> matter of fact, I must have been pretty good at it
> because Victory hired me for this eight months
> before I retired from the army.
> Interviewer: Since you had all that experience in the
> army, Victory hired you to set up new systems?
> Manager: Yes. One of the first things I did when I
> came here was set up the bakery. This entailed
> formulating policies, planning work flows, and
> training individuals for the job.

TRAINING AND DEVELOPMENT

Once employees are hired, the processes of orientation, training, and development become important. At Victory, these processes were no better oriented toward innovation and change than were the selection procedures. For the most part training was technically and procedurally oriented, with little or no emphasis on the development of human capabilities that would reinforce change and innovation. In pharmacy, for example, the chief pharmacist reported that:

> My assistant does most of the orientation. As I men-
> tioned, we have the pharmacy interns and the pharmacy
> students from the university. However, we don't have
> a formal program. We have a policy and procedures
> manual and this is available at all times and is part of
> the orientation program. . . .

And in the department of inhalation therapy, the director stated that orientation was procedural and was delegated to the night supervisor where new employees begin their work:

I have a policy of hiring only experienced inhalation
therapists. Because the work is very routinized,
an inhalation therapist can easily come in from another hospital and work here. However, when a new
employee does come to work for me, I put him on the
night shift and the night supervisor takes care of
orienting the new employees. There is a problem
occasionally where a new employee will be used to
doing a procedure one way at his former hospital
and has to learn to do the procedure a different way.

The training function was more highly developed in nursing
than anywhere else in the hospital, as would be expected in a professional group. The position of assistant director of staff education, directly subordinate to Winters, reflected the emphasis in
this area. The assistant director described her job as follows:

I'm in charge of planning and implementing programs
for continuing education for all personnel in the hospital, planning and supervising orientations for all
other personnel in the hospital, and I'm primarily
responsible for planning, implementing, and evaluating
plans for new unit-related educational programs, as,
for example, in medical intensive care.

In effect, the assistant director for staff education in the
nursing department fulfilled a staff training function that in many
organizations is administered within a centralized personnel department. Here is an account of a unit coordinator on one of the
nursing floors, also performing the training function as a line
manager:

In addition to my regular duties, I am responsible
for the planning, teaching, and in-service training.
This is done with the aid of staff education. Part of
the in-service training is in-the-unit teaching and I
have delegated this to the assistant unit coordinator,
along with the orientation of new personnel. I feel
that I can't do all this myself and therefore I have to
delegate certain responsibilities.

Several department heads indicated that the capability and
motivation to learn were important to them. This was especially
the case in the technical specialties where changes are frequent.
The neurosciences lab was one of the few units that recognized the

importance of personnel selection for innovation. According to the director:

> We have to be very selective. We're selective to the
> extent that we look for potential employees that are
> interested and want to learn. The reason is the par-
> ticularly unique problems in this field. One is that
> the work can be monotonous, routine, and exacting.
> Another problem, because of the interest of re-
> searchers in the field of neurology, is that there is
> a lot of technology generated. Therefore, the field
> as it affects the technicians is always changing. And
> the procedures are always changing. That is, they
> are becoming more complicated and sophisticated.

MANPOWER CONTROLS

Due to the absence of a strong, centralized personnel department at Victory, the higher administrators themselves maintained
tight controls over staffing, mainly through budgeting, financial,
and record-keeping methods. The manpower control process entailed substantial paperwork that many department heads felt was
unproductive. For example, the chief radiological technician
stated that:

> We don't have a shortage of technicians. However,
> the administration watches staffing very closely.
> When we have a resignation from the staff, they wait
> three or four weeks to replace him and save a little
> money. This area, for example, now has three people
> but it needs four. . . . Administration really watches
> numbers. They keep us on the borderline all the time
> on personnel. . . .

Even where extensive records on people were not kept, close
supervision provided strong controls over people. The manager of
the business office, for example, reported that:

> I don't keep extensive individual records. . . . I do
> randomly observe my employees to make sure they
> are working and I move around in the department
> and keep my eye on everybody. I feel that I would
> be wasting my time trying to gather information to
> set standards for my employees because I already
> know who is working and who is not.

Sometimes the manpower controls, going by figures in staffing reports, operated in a way that department heads thought were unfair. According to the chief radiological technician, defensive action is called for:

> We're watched very closely by administration. We have a man-hour budget and our money budgets. We try to be reasonable in asking for man-hours but we often run into problems. For example, here is a report showing that last August we had 200 overtime hours. Mr. Ellis has written on here "Too big" and sent it back to me. Now I've got to figure out how to show him that this hasn't been unreasonable. Now I've got to get some more facts, but I think I can show how this came about and why it was hard to avoid and why it is logical. See, there aren't many technicians in town. It's hard to get anybody to just come in and take somebody's place. So when somebody is sick or goes on vacation we have a lot of overtime.

The significance of tight controls of innovation and change lies in their effects on the attitudes of managers and their subordinates. While it is clear that cost problems in hospitals necessitate careful manpower control procedures, it should also be noted that tight controls may lower morale, and hence be an inhibiting factor for innovation and change. However, these inhibitions are due to manpower control and may be partly offset if they are examined in relation to output. According to Wright, high occupancy rates not only help maintain high morale but also point to the need for better manpower planning.

> Interviewer: One problem I have been looking to is the assertion that the ability to be creative depends on organizational slack, and that the best measurement of organizational slack is the occupancy rate in the hospital. What do you think?
>
> Wright: I think the organizational slack concept is valid. . . . First you have to remember that people in an organization don't sit idle. They will hide or make work unless they are fully assigned. Occupancy rates in a hospital and efficiency are on the same curve. That curve slopes upward and to the right until you are in the 90s and then it drops almost completely. . . . Beyond that 90 percent point, you are going to run into an impact on the physicians and the new patients. For example,

there are constraints on the assignment of beds
and rooms. First you have specialization by
floors, and then you have male or female problems, and then you have the heavy smokers and
so forth. Also, people want to be by the window
side. So when a patient asks for a change of beds
it can throw a lot of monkey wrenches into the
works. Also, there is a great deal of anger, emo-
tion, and frustration that comes into play. You
can't always use the second bed in a two-bed room
because of the condition of the patient. He might
smell bad or be too noisy or be a heavy smoker.
Now when you change a patient from one room to
another you've got to change all the records, his
name tag, the medical charts, and it is not as
simple as the patient thinks it is. So the only
meaningful way to handle occupancy is in its relationships to staffing. Your occupancy rate is
going up and down, 75 to 90 and back to 70 and up
to 95 again. With that variation you are going to
have a great deal of slack at certain times. There
is an excess of staff with wasted time and lost mo-
tion. High occupancy is O.K. but not beyond the
peak. At the peak, 90 percent of everything is in
a state of delicate balance. So what we work on is
the relationships of total employees to potential
work loads. The relationship of available personnel compared to the amount of work is better than
the census alone for a measure of organizational
slack. The way you put it, you assume that all
slack is the same and if that is true, then you are
right. High morale attracts the best people, and
when you have a high census, people get a sense of
accomplishment. They like the activity that is going on and it leads them to patterns of creativity.

We have examined how Victory Hospital manages the various
human capabilities that promote or impede innovation and change.
Personnel management at Victory, as in many hospitals, is largely
a province of the line. Although deprived of the presence of professional personnel administrators to serve as agents of innovation,
change, and development, Victory recognized the importance of
drawing upon available human capabilities that extend beyond the
merely technical. And although this part of the administrative environment is highly bureaucratic in its orientation toward strong

controls, the bureaucracy is managed in such a way as to hold and maintain a level of values, beliefs, attitudes, and morale conducive to innovation and change. In the next chapter we shall consider the processes of ideation, expectations, and the initiation of change innovation.

NOTES

1. Larry L. Cummings, Bernard L. Hinton, and Bruce P. Gobdel, "Creative Behavior as a Function of Task Environment: Impact of Objectives, Procedures, and Controls," Academy of Management Journal 18, no. 3 (September 1975): 489-99.

2. Salvadore R. Maddi, "Creativity Is Strenuous," University of Chicago Magazine, September/October 1973, pp. 18-23.

3. Ronald G. Corwin, "Strategies for Organizational Innovation," American Sociological Review 37 (August 1972): 441-54.

4. See, for example, psychoanalytical treatments by George Pickering, The Creative Malady (New York: Oxford University Press, 1975); and Rollo May, The Courage to Create (New York: Norton, 1975).

5. Warren G. Bennis, ed., American Bureaucracy (New Brunswick, N.J.: Transaction Books, 1970), Ch. 5.

6. Kenneth E. Knight, "A Descriptive Model of the Intra-firm Innovation Process," Journal of Business 40 (October 1967): 481.

7. Chris Argyris, Organizations and Innovations (Homewood, Ill.: Irwin-Dorsey Press, 1965).

8. Jon L. Pierce and André L. Delbecq, "Organization Structure, Individual Attitudes, and Innovation," Academy of Management Review, January 1977, p. 30.

9. R. D. Mytinger, Innovation in Local Health Services (Arlington, Va.: Public Health Service, Division of Medical Care Administration, U.S. Department of Health, Education and Welfare, 1968); L. B. Mohr, "Determinants of Innovation in Organizations," American Political Science Review (1969): 111-26.

10. A. Kaluzny, J. Veney, and J. Gentry, "Innovation of Health Services: A Comparative Study of Hospitals and Health Departments," MMFQ Health and Society 52 (Winter 1974): 51-82.

11. Pierce and Delbecq, op. cit., p. 33.

6

IDEATION, EXPECTATIONS, AND INITIATION

Traditional models of the innovation and change process begin with initiation, followed by adoption and implementation stages. However, in this study, it was found that a two-dimensional feedback model, shown in Figure 1.3, permits a more incisive analysis than the traditional linear stages model.

In the recommended model, initiation is preceded by ideation, managerial expectations, human capabilities, and the organizational context, as shown in Figure 6.1. The organizational context was examined in Chapters 3 and 4. Chapter 5 examined the capabilities of people. This chapter presents the findings with respect to ideation, expectations, and initiation.

IDEATION

Ideation is the term used in this study to describe the discovery, formation, and proposing of ideas within the organizational framework. This concept of ideation is somewhat broader than the dictionary definition: the capacity for the act of forming or entertaining ideas. It includes not only the surfacing of ideas for innovation and change and the manner in which an organization originates and then copes with ideas but also the perceptions of managers about the idea formation process and about the fate of ideas that arise.

The literature on innovation and change seldom treats ideation as such, although creativity is widely discussed. Most members of an organization, in the natural course of events, will produce a stream of more or less original ideas related to the tasks they perform. To the extent that such ideas are welcomed or at least not discouraged, they work their way in to the established ways of doing

FIGURE 6.1

Partial Model Showing Relationship of Key Factors
in Innovation and Change Up to and
Including Initiation

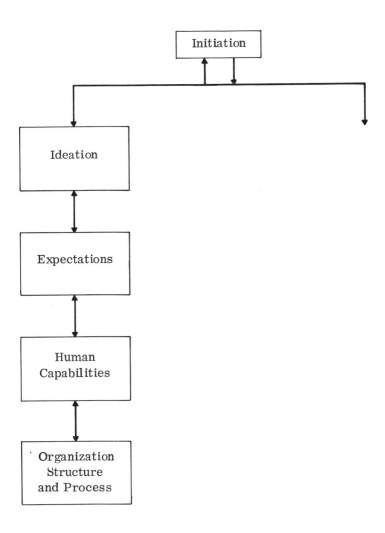

Source: Constructed by the author.

things. Some organizations, such as an advertising agency or a research and development firm, are deliberately designed to produce and cope with ideas.

High-technology industries and large complex or growing organizations, such as the metropolitan hospital, have high rates of technological innovation and change which have an impact on managerial innovation and change. The relatively abundant ideation found in Victory Hospital was in no small measure related to its size, growth, complexity, and high-technology characteristics. Yet one of the most significant forces producing ideas at Victory was the fact that its top administrators perceived the organization as an open, adaptive system alert for opportunities and change.

Pierce and Delbecq, in their summary of research and theory, found many inferences that organic (adaptive) organizations are innovative, that organizations with nonroutine tasks have high levels of innovation as product (or service) goals, and that decentralization is a primary predictor of innovation. The presence of individual and work unit autonomy, with less restricted communication flows, contributes to initiation activity in open organizations, and participative approaches in such organizations generates greater ego involvement and ultimate commitment to change, thus facilitating implementation.[1]

While Victory Hospital was structured bureaucratically, the expectations and perceptions of the top administrators reflected open-system behavior patterns, leading to high levels of ideation and initiation, as Pierce and Delbecq suggest. An examination of the sources of ideas and of managerial attitudes and expectations concerning ideation will affirm the importance of open-system characteristics if innovation is to be encouraged.

AMBIGUITY AND IDEATION

The first finding to be examined is that substantial ambiguity surrounds the ideation process. Rewards ordinarily do not go to the originators of ideas; they go to those who execute them, those who accomplish tasks and results. Those who implement ideas are usually not those who originate them. So much happens later in the innovation process that the earlier stage—ideation—becomes obscure.

By their very nature, ideas are elusive. Thoughts do not appear until they are manifest in some communication or are confirmed by changes in the behavior of people. A hidden resource in every organization is the welter of ideas dormant in the minds of its members. Under favorable conditions, individuals draw upon their thought processes to improve task performance, to benefit their personal situation, or to contribute to the organization's goals. Under risky or uninspiring conditions, individuals may hide or discard ideas without communicating or trying them. Thus, ideas may be examined according to whether they are localized, benefiting mainly the individual, or whether they can be generalized to other parts of the organization or to its total strategy.

The exact sources of adopted ideas were often hard to trace because interviewees often could not relate them to individual originators. None saw credit-grabbing as a problem, and as the time of an idea's use lengthened, its origins seemed to fade in the minds of the organization's members. This fading appeared to be associated with group acceptance and application. According to the vice president of business administration:

> . . . it is possible that some ideas come from young geniuses, from individuals. I think a more typical thing is that ideas just seem to evolve and you don't know which individual should get the credit. We get a lot of consensus in our group activities and before we know it we have some new thing to put into effect. I think it's more from the evolving situation than from particular individuals. None of us has time to sit around and think. Ideas come from working on real problems.

Another example of the fading of idea origination occurred in the physical therapy department. A new booklet was prepared describing therapies for certain specific disorders. The booklet was designed to improve communication between therapists and physicians. Asked where the idea came from, the director of physical therapy said:

> I think it was a group thing in that we all thought that it would be good for the department. However, I believe one of the girls brought in a booklet that was originally published somewhere else. When we reprinted it under our own name we gave the publisher and author credit. As I mentioned, it was a group thing. We all agreed that it would be good for doctors' information and also it would make the department look organized when people came around for accreditation. The booklet was particularly useful for another reason. . . . I felt this semblance of order would offset our poor showing in other administrative areas.

Two additional examples will serve to illustrate the ambiguities associated with the sources of ideas. Early in 1975, an employee call line was instituted. Employees can dial a number to make suggestions, comments, or complaints, or ask questions. In two months over 150 calls were made. Asked where the idea came from, Ellis said, "I don't know who thought of it. It may have come from some meeting . . . but nobody knows who first thought it up." But then he added:

> Now that I think of it the idea might have come from the
> personnel department at the central office. But I think
> it's more likely that they got the idea from one of our
> labor consultants who's been telling them things to do
> because of the union pressure we have been getting
> lately.

A color coding system was introduced in Victory's main building when it first opened. Each of the four wings of the building has its own identifying color to denote its equipment, documents, and other properties. According to the vice president of nursing:

> Nobody remembers what particular person thought of
> it. However, the idea came from the unit clerks. They
> thought of color coding and the unit coordinator brought
> the idea to the bimonthly nurses' meeting. The idea
> went like wildfire because it met an obvious need. Also,
> it was free of emotions and people weren't threatened
> by a change like that.

Ambiguity may be partly accounted for by the fact that ideas entail risks, such as that of rejection, criticism, or misappropriation. Therefore, the originator benefits from ambiguity at the cost of not getting credited with an idea. Some organization members enjoy "planting seeds" while remaining anonymous. Working behind the scenes provides an illusion of power that need not face the test of personal backing.

The uncertainty of an idea's fate is also a contributing factor. It is logical to expect that some ideas remain dormant at least temporarily, finding no suitable outlets for expression. Other ideas remain localized, being primarily of value to an individual or at most a group. Still others have a broad significance for major parts of the organization and for the total organization. For an idea to progress from an individual's brain to a significant place among the changes and innovations, it must undergo a complex process which includes (1) identification and formulation, (2) a trial balloon stage, (3) assessment and evaluation internal to the individual or the originating group, and (4) acceptance and approval by others affected and by higher echelons in the organization.

At the idea stage, an individual does not necessarily make an orderly assessment of the four stages by which an idea progresses to adoption. The conceiver knows, however, that controversy often surrounds proposed reforms or changes, and that a potentially dramatic struggle may ensue if the idea is put forth. The idea may arouse expectations among beneficiaries out of proportion to the realities of the improvement. Instead of winning gratitude, the originator may be attacked by beneficiaries as well as adversaries. The originator may also end up with obligations to supporters whose purposes he does not share and with fleeting credit but lasting antagonisms. Still, there are so many specialties, interests, skills, and people in a complex organization that it is impossible to suppress new ideas entirely. [2]

To bring an idea out into the open, an individual determines its possible benefits to himself and to others and considers the possible penalties and problems the use of the idea may bring to him or others. If the idea is not to be discarded, the individual needs a strategy to prove the idea's value and to gain the support of peers, subordinates, and superiors in the organization. Ideas cannot long remain the personal property of an individual. Once they are brought into the open, an organizational apparatus is ready to work them over. To be carried to an implementation stage, an idea needs sponsors and evidence of possible gains from its use. For example, the vice president of business administration reported that:

> Ideas are coming out all the time. We get a lot of suggestions and plans. In our meetings we try to critique the ideas. An idea might be attacked. We explore all the implications. We get the thinking of those who are involved or whose work will be affected and we try to examine the consequences of the ideas for the hospital and for everybody concerned. Usually with any one change many people are affected. For example, when I started a new budget policy I discovered that there were 50 or 60 people who were going to be affected by it and I hadn't realized it before.

INTERNAL SOURCES

Formal mechanisms for finding, developing, and rewarding ideas were minimal at Victory. As noted earlier, there was an absence of formalized staff groups which many organizations use to generate and develop ideas. The effects of this policy on innovation and change were most notable in the area of personnel management. Without a strong, central professional personnel group inside the Victory organization, it was difficult to develop personnel policies that enhance innovation. As indicated in the previous chapter, for example, the criteria for selection and placement did not include an individual's potential for ideas and innovation. Although several vice presidents and department heads thought this an important criterion, there did not appear to be an acceptable way of giving weight to this factor.

Rather than hiring idea people as such, it was the practice at Victory to expect ideas from all employees, especially from managers. Wright himself set the example for ideation. According to one of the vice presidents:

> One big factor is that Bill himself forces motivation. He comes up with huge lists of ideas, some crazy and some not so crazy. Bill is restless if people aren't working on new things. He wants things jumping all the time and going ahead. My counterparts in other hospitals don't have a Bill Wright to help them. They are simply working to keep their operations going without screw-ups.

That organizational climate was widely regarded as highly receptive to new ideas is indicated by the following comments from managers at several levels:

> People don't rush to call ideas bad or stupid. We take a good look at all of them. We are very open to ideas around here.

> This is a very progressive hospital. People who work here always know where they stand in their field and with other people. The climate is really very good. For example, in nursing we have started programs that no other hospital has. . . .

> Once a person establishes himself or has success in innovating, he will be well received.

> My ideas are well accepted here. There is no problem with this at all.

I am motivated by the fact that there is always a way
to operate the hospital a little better. I'm always
thinking of how to improve our work.

The importance of listening to others in order to get their
ideas was expressed by a number of department heads. For example, the head of the maintenance department said:

I'll tell you quite simply, I always listen to my people.
I found when I was a young man working as a millwright
that I could learn a lot more by listening than I could by
talking. My managing techniques may be a little different than you've encountered before but I believe that if
someone has something to say he should have the opportunity to say it. When you get to where you won't let
people give suggestions and you won't listen to what
they say then they are not going to beat you over the
head to tell you you are doing something wrong or you
should be doing something another way. They're just
not going to talk to you. . . . If somebody thinks he's
smarter than you are then it's gonna keep you from
talking to him because you're gonna feel that they know
it all, or at least they think they do. . . . If you want to
get something out of a person, you have to work with that
person not over him. That's why . . . any employee
that works for me can walk right in and talk to me. In
other words, I'm at their disposal and easily accessible
to them. . . .

Despite these general attitudes of acceptance for people's ideas,
a number of constraints were evident in addition to the need for control discussed above. Some informants felt that the system was not
really as open as it looked. For example, the physician in charge
of the pathology laboratory indicated that:

When I first came here I was told, well not actually
told but I got the idea, to just be quiet for five years
and carry on. When the buildings got set up and the
big·items were taken care of, then the administrators
would go around the departments. "Your time will
come," they said. Well, it never came. The time
came to the squeaky wheels, but I don't feel I should
have to scream and rave and rant and froth at the
mouth to get something. There is another way to do
it, but I don't think it's too ethical. I could go around

and stir up the staff and have them complain and turn
a lot of people against the administration. It works
faster, and I have done it a time or two. But we
shouldn't have to do things that way. What we really
need is more central, long-range planning and the
involvement of all the people.

That the absence of formal mechanisms that encourage ideation
inhibited the ideation process is reflected in the policy against suggestion plans. Suggestion plans are not only a form of upward communication but they also couple ideation to a specific reward system
that includes both money and psychic or intrinsic reward. Suggestion plans also guarantee that ideas will get a hearing. The absence
of such a plan was due to Wright, who based his objections on costs
relative to benefits:

We don't have a suggestion system here. We made a
definite decision not to. We thought that such a plan
involves too much expensive time. You spend a lot of
time reviewing ideas and suggestions that come in and
you perhaps get only three or four that are useful. It
just didn't seem to work out.

Another inhibition often appeared as distrust of the open system, accompanied by the feeling of managers that they, not subordinates, must carry the burden of ideation. Following a pattern
similar to Wright's, for example, the vice president of nursing reported that:

I envision myself as having four primary duties that
include coordinating, planning, linking, and thinking.
I consider myself the chief coordinator in my department for all nursing practice. . . . Another of my
duties is planning for and facilitating change. . . .
I see as one of my primary duties that of coming up
with ideas. I feel there is a general tendency to maintain the status quo and therefore it is necessary to have
someone at a high level who has ideas about new ways
of doing things.

Physicians were considered to be a productive internal source
of ideas, but these, too, encountered limitations, chiefly on the
basis of the costs of implementation. According to Vice President
Ellis:

The most potent source of ideas, I think, is our medical staff. Physicians give us a lot of good ideas . . .
but their thinking has a certain twist to it. For example, they don't pay any attention to finance or problems like that. They're interested in solving medical
problems, patient care, and things like that. Sometimes it's hard to cope with all the ideas that come out
of that group.

And again, according to Ellis:

You'll find that in hospitals the medical staff is one of the
strongest elements in innovation. It's also the strongest
factor against innovation. It's both pro and con. The
medical staff is necessarily a guiding force. If they are
an aggressive and capable group they are going to sell
their ideas. Take radiology for an example. They have
a forward look—therapy groups less so. The radiology
group has the drive, rapport, and momentum that the
entire medical staff ought to have. If the medical staff
is aggressive, it gets credibility. They provide a lot
of alternatives and assistance, drive and guiding direction for the best alternative.

The chief administrator and the four vice presidents have all been
described as innovative, change-oriented managers. They were all
aware of specific innovative efforts of their own, but willing also to
give credit to subordinates for their ideas. Yet they were also sensitive to the difficulties inherent in technology, organization structure, and the limitations of people. This was most clearly shown in
reflections by Dale Ellis:

I would say that innovation in our group is only moder-
ate. The mix of our work is fairly restricted. It isn't
exciting. It has limited scope and capabilities for
doing new things are limited. We don't have much
organization below the department head level. We
have to scramble and compete for labor, and the labor
is low-pay. It's hard to attract people at these levels.
So most of our innovating comes at the department
head level. However, we've done some good things
internally, in a self-controlled way. If I and my maintenance director agree to something, it's O.K. We
can go ahead and do it on our own. For example, we
made a significant change in installing our biomedical

maintenance program. The plant engineer and one
electronics man and I worked it all out. It was the
plant engineer's idea. The idea was to service our
own monitors and other equipment. This group maintains most of our electronic equipment, patient contact stuff. This idea came about through individuals
interested in a problem. It was cost-savings innovation, but there was some expense in training and
recruiting our own people to do the work.

Ideas sometimes emerge from department heads or supervisors
that have had strong inputs from their subordinates. Here are two:

Director of Environmental Services: Generally speak-
ing, I come up with most of the ideas in this department. But I listen to my supervisors. They handle
the day-to-day problems.

Business Office Manager: One of the girls in the insurance department made a suggestion about changing the form that we send down to be key punched to
go into the computer file. The change amounted to
blocking out or deleting some of the requirements
from the key punch sheet because we already had the
information. This in effect saved her time.

On balance, internal sources provide a primary generating base
for ideas. Managers are aware of the organization's dependence on
people for innovative thinking, as well as the importance of the need
for ideas. The undercurrent of desire for order and control, as well
as the practical considerations of cost, yields interesting insights
for the management in respect to ideas and ideation. The principal
problem of innovation in Victory was not to get ideas heard. Rather,
difficulties came in later stages—adoption and implementation.
Later it will be shown that the absence of formal ideation mechanisms
and policies inhibits not only the ideation process but the adoption
and implementation phases as well.

OUTSIDE SOURCES

We have established that Victory's key managers viewed the
organization as an open system, even though strong elements of
bureaucracy were maintained. The real test of the extent to which
an organization is an open one is found in its relationships to the

external environment. In particular, it is vital to the dynamics of innovation and change that organizations monitor the external environment for ideas and other influences that promote the need for change and adaptation.

The relationships between a hospital and its task environment are created and maintained through a type of activity known as boundary spanning. That is, the organization's boundaries must be sufficiently open to allow two-way interaction and communication between its members and those of outside organizations or constituencies. Formal boundary spanning occurs when certain members have as their duty, all or in part, the exchange of information or the management of other transactions concerning people, ideas, money, or materials. Informal boundary spanning takes the form of interactive exchanges that occur indirectly by reason of the coming and going of organization members.

At this point we shall consider only those aspects of boundary spanning which relate to ideation. Outside sources, through boundary spanning behavior, provided many ideas which influenced internal decisions and actions at Victory. Three types of outside sources will be analyzed for their effects on ideation at Victory: (1) the use of outside consultants, (2) mandates and opportunities arising from public agencies, and (3) the travel and professional association activities of organization members.

It was indicated earlier that the use of outside consultants was extensive at Victory. Between 1973 and 1975, according to Wright, the consultants included a local firm for two studies, one of pathology procedures and one of physician effort; a firm from Ann Arbor doing a work standards study; an insurance consultant for pension and retirement programs; an architectural firm on building problems; a land use consultant for property development; Arthur Young, Inc., for job evaluation work; a labor consultant; a prominent general hospital consulting firm; an engineering consultant; and a number of individual consultants for attitude surveys, seminars, and training sessions. In addition, Wright viewed the hospital's part-time attorney as a consultant.

This piecemeal, ad hoc use of consultants reveals the lack of concerted attacks on major problems and of the development of an overall, integrative approach. This accounts in part for the fact that the resulting inputs of ideas and the amount of change induced by them were relatively small. Wright explained that much depends on the kind and difficulty of the problem given to a consultant:

> Wright: The value of outside consultants ranges all the way from 0 to 100 percent. With some, we never follow any of their advice and with others we wouldn't

deviate a bit. An example is the organization study
by a local firm. That study caused an awful lot of
trouble and difficulty, turmoil, and tribulation
around here and it was so disruptive that we finally
shelved it.

Interviewer: That seems to happen quite often?

Wright: There is one thing you should remember about
consultants. Whether you follow their recommenda-
tion or not they always have an impact. Even if you
don't follow their advice, they leave behind them a
lot of pressures, ideas, suggestions, opinions, and
the like. Their impact may be either negative or
positive, but it is always there.

Interviewer: Yes, but you don't hire a consultant for
that, do you? How can you improve your batting
average with consultants?

Wright: One of the primary factors in a consultant's
success is the motivation and commitment which the
organization has with respect to the problem he is
working on. We've had one extreme success, but as
I say, it is rare. . . . The organization should use
a great deal of care in selecting a consultant and most
of the time it doesn't. Then the organization isn't
really committed to support the consultant. Often we
aren't that involved while he's here. He may do some
interesting things and will tell us about them. He will
uncover some facts and principles and have some
things to say to us. But what are the personal outcomes? Is the manager willing to carry out his suggestions? Most of the time the answer is no.

The "extreme success" to which Wright referred in the above
comments was the Index-12 program under Ellis's direction. Ellis
was himself a product of extensive experience as a hospital consultant. He had an industrial engineering background, and Wright
had hired him from a prominent hospital consulting firm frequently
used by Victory. Ellis himself was by training a generator of ideas.
It was he who thought of the Index-12 program, which entails a systematic record and analysis system for manpower control. According to Ellis:

We did it right here, and not in the general office or at
Bright. It is a manpower control system that helps us
evaluate where we are and where we are going. It's a
valuable manpower planning tool that came out of my own

background as a consultant. I have put this idea into
effect in several places. We also had the help of a
consulting firm. Bill Wright called this "our biggest
success of 1974."

Despite his experience and perceptivity about consultants,
however, Ellis agreed with Wright that the batting average of consultants in bringing about successful change was low: "We have had
some outstanding successes, but this is pretty rare with an outside
consultant. Failures are more common than successes."

An example of an idea that did not work out occurred when a
consultant retained to study work standards made a suggestion that
was subjected to participatory decision making. According to Vice
President Watson, Victory hired the consultant to improve their
venapuncture blook collection work. They were dissatisfied with
the staff's results, so a consulting firm was retained to do an industrial engineering study for work measurement and establishment of
work standards. The consultants came up with the idea of a four-
day work week. He asked the people affected to think it over for
a week, and told them they could decide. They decided not to go
to the four-day week because they wouldn't like it, so Watson didn't
push it. He decided to try it again later because he didn't want to
force it on them.

An additional perspective on consultants as a source of ideation
came from an interview with the chief administrator at Victory's
sister hospital, Bright. He cited a tendency in the Norfield organization to utilize consultants in carrying out things to be done, rather
than helping to decide what to do:

We waste a lot of money on consultants and research.
We have them make studies of how to carry out things
rather than on whether to carry them out. Here at
Bright we do the opposite. We use them to test ideas,
not develop them. We know how to develop them but
we want to know if the idea is sound first. . . . We
need the consultants to give us guidelines and alternatives.

A second category of outside sources of ideation consist of the
linkages between the hospital and organizations in the public sector—
community agencies, coordinating boards, educational institutions,
licensing and accrediting agencies, inspectors, regulating bodies,
and many government agencies and bureaus. An enormous amount
of administrative and clinical time is required to meet these demands, but in many cases the outside forces become a factor in

managerial change. From the point of view of administrators and other hospital personnel such as physicians, ideas with wide public acceptance are forced into the organization by legislation aimed at public benefits, apart from internal considerations or analysis of their merits. In other words, a legally imposed idea for change moves rapidly into the implementation stage with virtually no adoption decision process. Thus, ideas of vital interest to hospitals are debated externally rather than internally and prior to rather than after they are actually introduced into the organization.

Professional Standards Review Organizations (PSROs) provide an example of the impact of outside political, economic, and social forces originating in the public sector. PSRO requirements, for example, forced Victory to create a new position entitled health record analyst. According to the analyst:

> My position as health record analyst is not only a new job but has sprung up because of a new need, the legislative act by Congress requiring a Professional Standards Review Organization. . . . This legislation has caused problems for certain hospitals. Some of the smaller ones are doing nothing to meet these problems and are in effect waiting for larger hospitals such as ours to set guidelines for them. We've realized the need to coordinate our efforts. One way administration felt it could accomplish this was to put someone with age and experience in this new position.

Similar pressures were also felt in nursing, where a new system of audit evaluations for nursing services was instituted. According to the director of nursing:

> Audit evaluations reveal the activities and standards of our nursing practices. There's a lot of pressure for audit evaluations. You've got your PSROs and other things like that putting demands on professional people like the doctors. The same thing is happening in nursing. We need to work on better criteria and higher standards. That's for both doctors and nurses. It ought to be possible to fuse them and bring them together. Doctors and nurses ought to get together more, but there is no such thing as a team between doctors and nursing administrators. I know you hear there is, but there is cooperation, not a team. We would be the first to try the impossible, but without progress you soon lose hope. It isn't an original

idea with me. I've heard it said in meetings nationally that we should forget teamwork, that it's too idealistic a concept.

Hospital personnel generally reacte to PSRO regulations as inevitable but a source of difficulties. Physicians were negative in their views, chiefly because of the increased complexity it brings to their decision processes. According to one physician:

Nobody likes it. It's going to take a lot more time and effort on the part of the medical people to fulfill the requirements. The way things have been working until now hasn't been too bad. When we had an argument with Blue Cross or somebody on whether a patient who had stayed seven days should only have stayed five days and they won't pay for the other two days, our executive committee has looked into it and they could readily solve the problem. . . . Under the PSRO system there are a lot more complications.

The chief health record analyst also expressed the difficulties of carrying out PSRO regulations:

The law says that hospitals have the choice of either setting criteria for patients being admitted to hospitals and patient services or that the government will set the criteria. Presently, I'm working with the doctors and the staff trying to develop the criteria. . . . Actually, there are two ways we can go about it—the concurrent review or the retrospective review. The concurrent review involves looking at the criteria we've developed and then looking at the present maintenance of patients who are in house and see if there's any necessary or unnecessary variation. The retrospective review involves looking at the criteria and then looking at the data that we abstract on patients and comparing the variances. If we can justify the variances by legitimate reasons, then there is no problem. However, the government has made it clear that it is not going to pay for custodial care. There are three problems that seem to show up more than others when we evaluate the abstracts: (1) lack of equipment, (2) work just wasn't done, or (3) knowledge or performance problems of the doctors. Let me explain that last one. We may have to keep a patient in the hospital longer because the

doctor may lack some skill, he may be behind in his
reading, or it may only be an idiosyncrasy. When
and if we find these problems, we would ordinarily
go to the department for corrective action. Actually,
I believe the government has become so tight about
this problem mainly because the 100-bed or less hospitals with occupancy problems keep patients in longer
than they should just to generate additional revenue.
For hospitals such as this, 1976 is the end of the line.
The government has said if you don't establish a review mechanism of your own, it will and if you don't
conform the claims will be denied.

Pressures and conflict were found to be a major factor in the
impact of ideas from outside sources. PSRO requirements were
instituted by the threat of withdrawal of Medicare and Medicaid
payments. To illustrate further, an analyst in the business office
indicated similar pressure of this type:

Most of the changes that have affected us from outside
have been deleterious. For example, we were informed that on July 1 the Medicare program would
institute a new form called a Reply to Notice of Admission. Whenever we admit anyone who qualifies
for Medicare or Medicaid we have to submit this
form to Medicare and they tell us whether we should
charge the patient or the Medicare program. . . .
With 25 percent of the patient census on Medicare,
these individuals represent a substantial amount of
revenue for the hospital. We weren't allowed to
process the billing of these Medicare patients until
the reply to Notice of Admission was received. But
after July 1 we didn't get any notices back, so we were
backlogged about a month on our billings.

Another type of internal pressure arises from service demands.
These were expressed by Victory's chaplain as follows:

A lot depends on the purpose and intent of the organization. That has a lot to do with creativity. You have to
intend to be creative and innovative. . . . I also think
pressure and demands for service give a strong motivation for creativity and innovation. All aspects of a hospital have some religious values associated with them.
For example, there is the old-fashioned biblical idea of

stewardship, and the value we attribute to humans. If we follow some of these precepts you'll get innovation and creativity.

Conflict provides another internal source of pressure for generating ideas and innovation. A keen observer, one of the management interns, described the administrative executive committee as the main source of innovation at Victory. He felt that conflict and tension are instrumental in moving ideas from one locus to another in complex patterns of interaction, but that the top administrators resolve conflicts through innovative actions:

> Interviewer: Could you develop the idea of the committee a little?
> Intern: Yes. Hospitals work on what is called a conflict theory. That is, as needs or pressure points arise, the administrative organization or the staff members react to lessen the pressure of the conflict or the need. But there's really not much going on if there is not much need. In other words, there's a correlation there between pressures and innovation.
> Interviewer: Can you give me an example of how your conflict theory works?
> Intern: O.K. The job posting system is employed by many hospitals to combat the effects of dead-end jobs—where employees cannot go any higher or make any more money. . . . The system tends to give preference to employees who meet the qualifications for the jobs, as opposed to bringing in new blood from outside. . . . But the committee has to deal with the employees and the unions that have been holding up this change. I think in time it's going to get implemented.

The director of environmental services reported initiating the job posting idea by first establishing such a system in her department. Eventually the personnel department started a general posting system where the directors of each department sent their job notices to personnel for posting in a central location.

A third major outside source of ideation came from the influence of various associations, boards, or other organizations with which either individuals or the hospital itself maintains relationships. For example, architects and designers are shifting to the belief that single-person rooms are better for patients, thereby influencing expansion and construction of new buildings.

Educational activities also play a role in ideation. For example, Victory had close ties with a nearby university medical school. It continuously utilized a number of management interns taking their degrees in hospital management. Interns are assigned to projects and studies of the type usually assigned to staff departments or to task forces. For example, one was assigned to work on Victory's part of a national nursing evaluation study and Victory's pension and employee benefit programs.

There were also many interns from technical schools. Victory's department of inhalation therapy found it necessary to respond to the demands of the accrediting agency for one of the schools from which it drew interns. The department had no formal medical committee to advise on medical matters. A nearby school of inhalation therapy was required by its accrediting agency to place student interns only where the hospital's department had such a committee. Threatened by withdrawal of the interns, a medical committee was established, permitted continuation of the internships, and, in addition, solved a problem for the department by providing direct access to medical advice. The students were highly prized by the director of inhalation therapy for their ideas as well as for their labor.

Finally, some examples of the ideation process in the form of boundary spanning will show that this is a vital source of ideas. One example is provided by the head of the neurosciences laboratory:

> Technological innovations come from doctors and researchers, of course. However, the ideas filter down to us through two main bodies or societies. One is a society of doctors called the American Encephalogram Society. Another, is the society for neuroscience technicians called the Society of Electroencephalograph Technicians. These two groups are very close and have joint conventions and meeting privileges. . . . The ideas come through both societies in the form of monthly periodicals and annual conventions for each.

It would be naive to proclaim that large numbers of ideas produced at association meetings and obtained from journals are put into action or that they receive automatic adoption. Quite the contrary. Ideas from these sources were scrutinized as carefully as ideas produced internally. But would-be change agents received reinforcement from hearing the experiences of others, and ammunition for the persuasion process. Thus it may take considerable time for an idea to make its way through the organizational processes to its ultimate use. One informant, for example, reported

a four-year interval during which extensive work was done to secure acceptance. The director of the pathology laboratory attended
a conference that dealt with some new ideas about audit review
committees to one committee for all reviewing. However, the
director reported that:

> Yes, I brought back the idea but I wasn't the first one.
> Our people have been going to that conference for the
> past four years and have been coming back with ideas,
> but I guess this was an idea whose time had come and
> I was the last one to come back and bring it up again,
> so I get the credit.

And, according to one of the physicians on the medical staff:

> I think we're better than average at innovation. We have
> a lot of people who are interested in ideas. We have
> good administrators. They travel a lot, they get around
> and see what ideas are going on. And they have money.
> Having capable administrators and having money is good
> for innovation. They get around enough to see how new
> ideas work somewhere else, and then we can try them
> out here. Our board members spend a lot of time look-
> ing at new ideas too. They go out on trips and get around
> and they are very receptive to change and innovation.

Vice President Ben Watson also indicated the value of outside sources:

> Interviewer: Where do most of the good ideas come
>   from here?
> Watson: Well, my colleagues and I go to a lot of
>   meetings. We read all the literature coming out,
>   and we attend conferences around the country with
>   our peers from outside. We get quite an informa-
>   tion input from this kind of activity.

And, according to the vice president of nursing, herself a frequent
traveler:

> We send people away a lot—our chief nurses or our unit
> coordinators or their assistants. We send them around
> visiting hospitals; they see new ideas and bring them
> back in and we talk about them and try them out. A lot
> of us keep going to meetings and we get a lot of good
> ideas that way.

We have shown in this chapter a number of vital internal and external forces that generate ideas in Victory Hospital. Many ideas arise in the minds of people who are trying to improve their work. Others arise from problem solving. Still others are thrust upon the organization by powerful outside forces in the form of technological development, patient needs and demands, socioeconomic and political pressures, the omnipresence of local, state, and federal regulations, and authentication of boundary spanners responding to influences from professional associations and accrediting agencies. Conflict and the pressures of accreditation affect the generation, shaping, and use of ideas.

In the following chapter, we turn to a more detailed examination of several categories of change and the processes by which ideas are transformed into change.

NOTES

1. Jon L. Pierce and André L. Delbecq, "Organization Structure, Individual Attitudes, and Innovation," Academy of Management Review, January 1977, pp. 30-31.

2. Herbert Kaufman, The Limits of Organizational Change (University: University of Alabama Press, 1971), pp. 14, 22.

7

PLANS, STRATEGIES, AND CHANGE

Following the model presented in Chapter 1, we have considered the elements of the innovation process which lead to initiation: organization structure and process, human capabilities, expectations, and ideation. Our next task is to examine the plans and strategies which persuade organization members to move into the adoption stage. This part of the model is shown in Figure 7.1.

Based on their survey of research findings, Pierce and Delbecq advance two propositions relevant to this part of our inquiry: (1) Environmental uncertainty will be positively related to organizational innovation (initiation, adoption, and implementation). (2) The values of strategic decision makers favorable toward change will be positively related to organizational innovation.[1]

The studies at Victory and similar hospitals give general support to both propositions. Evidence for the influence of strategic decision makers was presented in earlier chapters. However, these propositions highlight the planning functions of administrators. Accordingly, this chapter reviews the processes of planning for change and the relevant beliefs of Victory's managers in order to provide further insights about the relevance of the propositions.

The reality of change as a way of life at Victory Hospital was widely accepted at all levels of the organization. This awareness of omnipresent change, however, was coupled with sensitivity toward the difficulties and complexities of both inevitable change and desirable change. The pace and extent of change was reported to be high by nearly all managers interviewed. A typical statement was that "We change so fast around here I can't keep track of things. . . ."

FIGURE 7.1

Partial Model Showing Relationships of Plans, Strategies, and Persuasion to Preceding Elements of the Total Model

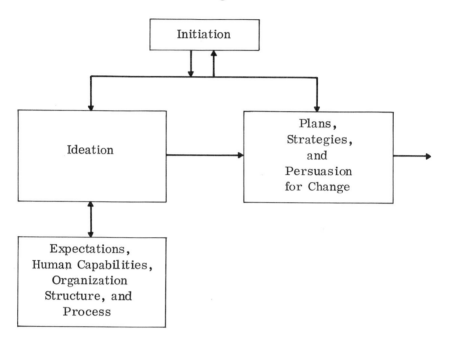

Source: Constructed by the author.

PLANNING FOR CHANGE

The substantial change consciousness among the administrators at all levels at Victory Hospital was reflected in restlessness or dissatisfaction with existing conditions and in their knowledge of trends and ideas in the hospital field generally. Planning activity was modeled for Victory by the actions and policies of the top management group at Norfield. Leonard Hayfield, Norfield's vice president for finance, expressed the planning viewpoint:

> We have a lot of things happening. The board of trustees, in spite of all our staffing problems, has expressed its intentions to keep going and keep going well. They still have their overall objective of finding the best ways of serving the community and the

patients. It isn't just growth and expansion for expansion's sake. They have definite objectives in mind. We are entering into some new affiliations, and that's part of the plan to expand our community service.

Hayfield also described several plans for change that would substantially affect both Victory and Bright Hospitals:

Right now I'm working on a $25,000,000 bond issue. . . . Another thing we're going to do is combine Bright and Victory into a single corporation in order to get more significant coordination. . . . Mr. Wright and the administrator at Bright get along pretty well together and there is a lot of cooperation. However, each one naturally tends to think of his own unit first. Each one wants to get something out of it. . . . They can't be expected to enter into coordinated arrangements just for the sake of it, or just because the central office here might want it. They have to see what they gain by it first. With the separate corporations, we don't have an easy time with this end of things. Besides, combining the corporations will assist us in the bond issue we are putting through.

The commitment of Victory's managers to planning was revealed by statements in annual reports and other documents. With few exceptions, the reports of vice presidents and department heads indicated plans in progress as well as changes being contemplated. For example, at Victory, there were extensive plans for reorganizing the personnel function. Documents disclosed that in 1974 plans were being worked on to (1) completely reorganize the personnel functions at Victory and the central office, (2) relocate the personnel office from the Victory building to the adjacent Professional Office Building, (3) set up a new position for a director of employee training, (4) set up a personnel information retrieval system, and (5) implement a new hospital-wide system of job posting.

Victory was also considering a plan to construct a new unit to house all three of its intensive care units. This building would be part of the main building but would contain all intensive care services (coronary, surgical, and medical care) in a cohesive unit. And Winters, the vice president of nursing, planned to enlarge the corps of nursing specialists by two additions in 1975: a research nurse with a Ph.D. in nursing research and a specialist nurse with a master's degree in medical-surgical training.

A primary prerequisite for substantial successful innovation and change is the careful planning and analysis undertaken before major changes are made. According to Wright, "We are making operating studies here all the time." One of the primary tasks assigned to management interns is to make studies of specific problems in preparation for anticipated change. In 1974, for example, one of the management interns was doing research on (1) the evaluation of nursing performance, (2) an information dissemination system to communicate to employees the value and scope of their fringe benefits, and (3) a project to study the feasibility of a "cafeteria system" of employee benefits, where the hospital would allow each employee to choose his own benefit mix within a fixed dollar amount.

Systematic planning was important to Wright, who conducted his working relationships with the vice presidents on an informal management by objectives (MBO) concept which involved careful goal planning on their part. The vice presidents used similar methods. Ellis described this process as follows:

> My departments work by annual objectives. It's not the classic MBO program, but something like it. I work with each of my department heads to set the goals for the next year. We talk about operating problems and about desired improvements. We don't talk about vague missions; we get right down to brass tacks. For example, our housekeeping had gone to hell and we wanted to improve it. Using my engineering background, I helped them analyze the problem and we found that it was scheduling. We introduced the use of Gantt charts. This helped a lot, but the department heads tend to ignore the charts and I have to keep after them to get them to do it. This goal planning is new in our group. Some earlier efforts failed, probably because things were too vague. They never came up with a real action plan. The way we do it now leads to actual budget impacts.

Ellis utilized predominantly a one-to-one planning approach with each department head, feeling that the group had not matured to the point of being ready for group planning. By contrast, planning in several units followed a group approach. Physicians in the radiology laboratory, for example, followed a long-range group process, according to the physician in charge:

We are always planning three to five years ahead. This
is a good policy for our group and also for the hospital.
We first develop our plans financially. In some organizations, finance drives the planning. That's not so with us.
We plan first, then try to get the money. We plan what's
best for patients, try to cut cost by speed, and emphasize
quantity and quality. We all do a lot of traveling to meetings. That way we hear about new things and we compare
them to our needs and over a five-year period can do
some planning.

In the nursing education function, the director also followed
group strategies:

Interviewer: How do you zero in on the most important
aspects of a new program?
Director: By means of cooperation among the staff in
my department. We decide what priorities are important in a program and choose a format. In this
way we make a group effort to establish teaching
policies and guidelines.
Interviewer: It's a kind of group process?
Director: Yes. That is an accurate description. Each
fall we lay out an annual plan which describes our
hopes and expectations for the coming year. Of
course other things are inserted during the year and
therefore we must have a flexible plan.

One aspect of the planning process that was vital in Victory was
the insistence on supporting plans for change with adequate data so
that administrators could be persuaded to approve them. For example, the chief radiological technician said that, "I would never
take any ideas to Mr. Wright without a plan of action." And concerning a plan to improve the productivity and reliability of workers
in the venapuncture blood collection group, one of the vice presidents
reported that:

We made a study of the problem. This group comes in
and works from 6 to 8 a.m. It is hard to get people to
work that early in the morning, but we need to do it.
The problem depends on how many admissions we have.
So we devised a system of paying them a fixed amount
for two hours of work. If they get the job done sooner,

they can go. If it takes them longer, they have to put the time in. We have to let these people make more money or we can't get them to come in early.

Another example of information search in planning for change was provided by Wright, the chief administrator, who wanted to develop Victory's outpatient services. He asked the medical record analyst to find information relevant to the problem:

Recently Mr. Wright gave me a list of surgical procedures and he wanted me to find out from doctors how many of them could be done on an outpatient basis. . . . Yesterday I showed this list to a doctor who is on our staff. He said he already did quite a few of them in his office. There is a real probability over the next two or three years that a 20 percent decrease in the hospital census nationally will result from this trend. We're going to have to be as imaginative as possible and figure out ways to do more surgery on an outpatient basis.

The planning processes at Victory appeared to be under vigorous direction by members of the top management group, but this occasionally was resisted by department heads, who resented the element of control. For example, the admitting department was involved in planning forecasts of the patient census on a daily basis. Here the planning system entailed parallel forecasts by the chief administrator, one of the operations vice presidents, the vice president for business administration, and the head of the admitting department. These multiple forecasts were then compared against the actual daily census. The head of admitting disliked forecasting and made an unsuccessful attempt to eliminate it:

I think administration watches our planning very closely. Once I tried to eliminate forecasting completely and administration became very upset. Both Mr. Wright and Mr. Watson have their secretaries estimate a daily census and then compare it against mine. Also, Mrs. Nelling compiles a forecast for her own financial purposes and it's interesting to see who is more accurate.

Planning also was found upon occasion to be meaningless where the department head, by temperament, did not pursue the plans that the group developed. A nurse, for example, reported that the director of nursing education made the group determine goals and plans, "but would never let us complete them. She kept us busy just putting out fires."

From the foregoing analysis, it is clear that planning occupied a great deal of administrative attention. By definition, planning represents a concern for the future and implicitly recognizes the value of orderly change. We will now examine a number of important changes that occurred at Victory in order to show the influences that the task environment brought to the administrators and managers.

CHANGE PROCESSES AT VICTORY

The proposition that environmental uncertainty is positively related to innovation reflected the impact of conditions external to the system of internal functioning. The hospital's task environment is generated by patients, physicians, competitors, suppliers, regulatory bodies, and scientific, technical, and professional reference groups. The different units of the hospital are affected in different ways by particular task environment influences, but all must deal the best they can, through planning and change decisions, with the uncertainty pervading their task environments.

Purely discretionary changes are few in number and tend to relate to internal operating problems, such as improving procedures. Even here, however, many of the ideas come from external environments, through linkages and contacts with task-related agencies, individuals, or associations. Moreover, the task environment of one unit may involve interrelationships with the other units it is designed to serve or which serve it. These linkages involve a service orientation, and service to an internal or external clientele rationalizes a great deal of change and innovation.

The initiating force of the service orientation is illustrated by a comment of the head of the department of inhalation therapy:

> I do know that this is a changing new service and it can be explained for two reasons. One is that inhalation therapy is a vital service to the welfare of the patient, and doctors have begun to realize this and demanded our services. We've had to grow and we've had to change. Another reason is that our department is a revenue producer, that is, for every dollar spent in inhalation therapy, we make four dollars.

An organizational change with respect to inhalation therapy affected the nurses because it removed one of their functions, and in addition, led to the problem of a shortage of space. In 1966, when Victory opened at its new location, RNs were giving inhalation therapy. By 1973, a new and separate department was established, transferring the work from nurses to technical specialists. However, when the hospital was designed and built, there was no space allotted to inhalation therapy because in 1966 RNs were responsible for administering the therapy. Subsequently, a space shortage remained.

To illustrate further, changes in the pharmacy had great impact on nursing and radiology as well as on patients. The radiology department, for example, benefited by the movement of the pharmacy from the first to the second floor. According to Ellis: "It had a hell of an impact on radiology because they got the space on the first floor that the pharmacy moved out of. Radiology is expanding a lot. Now they are getting ready to take angiographs and tomographs. . . ."

Another change in the pharmacy that affected both patients and nurses was the adoption of a new patient profile system. One of the pharmacists described this change as follows:

> With this new system we use the drug order from the doctor in his own handwriting. By getting the original, we cut down on the amount of human error that used to be involved in transcribing the orders for nurses. Basically, the system entails a more logical processing of the orders as we get them from the floors with more control and safeguards built into the system. What happens is we get the original order from the doctor and our profile clerk records it. Then the order is put on a profile chart to be filled. The pharmacist then fills the order and checks the order copy against the original. Then someone else, usually another pharmacist, checks the order. We feel that the three checks built into this system help minimize mistakes.

Many of the changes made by one group that affect other groups were at the policy rather than procedural or operational level. For example, the pharmacy introduced a new drug control system for the preparation of intravenous injections. According to the chief pharmacist:

> We have a new IV [intravenous] additive program that we are currently working on and plan to implement soon. The intravenous program would require pharmacists to mix drugs into IV fluids rather than nurses. Usually when a doctor orders an IV fluid, he also orders additives such as vitamins and potassium and other medications. . . . These additions are usually made by the

nurses on the wards. In the new program, the pharmacist rather than the nurse will make these additions under sterile conditions and high-quality control. The main advantages are that they are done under sterile techniques, it helps nurses and frees them to attend to the patient more, and it provides a quality control in that we have more precise measurement devices here in the pharmacy.

There were rarely changes made that did not affect other units and were intended to improve internal operations rather than patient care or the delivery of services. Instead of a service rationale, these types of change proceeded by an inner logic of their own. They would not occur without a managerial value system that rates efficiency of operations as worthwhile. In the admitting department, for example, the director's personal observations of work flow problems and attitudes toward work led to the change process:

I've made a lot of changes since I've been here simply by using rational thinking and asking myself why a certain procedure has to be institutionalized. For instance, when I took over as director I noticed that when a patient was admitted we made two addressograph cards. I couldn't understand why we needed two so one day I went along with the cards to see what they were used for. I saw that one of the cards went to the floor where the patient was located and from there it was put into a drawer and used only when medication was taken to a patient's room, or brought back and put in the drawer. I reasoned that a single cardboard card would be just as good as a plastic addressograph card and would save the department money by not having to make two. I found a lot of this kind of waste and inefficiency not only in my department but in others. It seems to me quite often that employees don't ask themselves why they are doing something—they just perpetuate inefficiency.

COMPUTERIZATION

Many internal changes at Victory involved contacts outside the organization, through planning and research, the services of outside consultants, and the knowledge of changes used elsewhere to improve efficiency, to lower costs, or to make work simpler and more logical.

The computerization effort at Victory further illustrates how an essentially internal change process is linked to outside influences. Computerization changed the task environment by reducing environmental uncertainty through better information processing and records management.

Computerization wrought extensive change throughout the Victory organization. It moved through several stages, all involving extensive planning. Prior to 1971, Victory shared a computer system with another large hospital in the same city. Because cost studies indicated substantial savings if Norfield had its own computer, in early 1971 an outside consulting firm was retained to establish and operate a computer system for the entire Norfield Complex. An IBM-360 was installed, with the basic equipment placed at Bright Hospital.

In 1975, the computer installation was changed from an IBM-360 to an IBM-370 system. The equipment was relocated to Norfield's new central office building. This process took over a year of planning and preparation, but it greatly expanded the application and use of the computer. By 1975, the areas of activity that were substantially computerized were admitting, personnel records, payroll, and several additional types of data processing and record keeping. According to Nelling, the vice president for business administration at Victory, "We have plans to put several other functions on an on-line basis later on so this is a big development effort for us." She indicated that she saw data collection as a prerequisite for innovation:

> At the moment my main concern is not with innovation.
> My main concern this year has been to provide good
> data collection. . . . Hospital people are noted for
> their lack of concern about data and it is hard to get
> them to provide it systematically. We have been
> forced to get more sophisticated data on man-hours,
> patient census, various counts, procedures, etc.
> The computer has both assisted us in doing this and
> forced us to do it. I first started working on budgetary
> problems, but weaknesses in the budget process showed
> the need for more and better data. So first I set up the
> mechanics, then I had to educate the system to use
> the data. Everything we do now is on computer. It
> has changed our entire way of life here.

How these changes affected one of Nelling's departments is illustrated by the way computerization changed the reporting system. According to the manager of the business office:

Since I became business manager, I have had to change
the format of some of my reports to Mrs. Nelling. . , .
By screening and deleting some of the information from
these reports, we saved a lot of time and effort. Another thing I have done is to concentrate more attention
throughout the department on the accuracy of billing. . . .
Finally, you probably noticed the cathode ray tube [CRT]
out in the office. . . . The CRT was part of a computerized program system that was implemented just before I
became manager. It gives Mrs. Nelling direct access to
the computer and to current information on patient accounts.

One early change made possible by the computer was an indexing system in the medical records section. This system combined
a disease index, a doctor's index, and an operations index into an
automated system called the Professional Activity Study. According
to the medical records director:

One day Mr. Wright asked me what I had heard about
Professional Activity Studies. I told him nothing good,
but I would see what I could find. I researched all the
available literature on the system. I found out that it
was good but that it had received a bad name because
certain individuals had been resistant to change. I'm
sure that after what I learned about the system that it's
going to be around for a long time, and as a matter of
fact it is the system of the future for this type of automated data.

The fact that record keeping and data processing are important
to the change process was also indicated by the supervisor of neurosciences:

My predecessor kept records, but not as extensively as
I do, I had to pick up where she left off and tailor-make
some things to fit my thinking. By keeping the kind of
records that I feel are pertinent, occasionally I can make
a study or rationalize making a change in the work flow.
For example, not long after I took over the department,
I changed and streamlined the procedure for processing
a patient. You wouldn't believe the way it used to be.
There seemed to be no rhyme or reason to the whole
thing. By designing a more comprehensive registration
form and modifying the work flow in the department

itself I made it not only easier on the patient but also
on the employee who was doing the work. We used to
admit one patient at a time and if this patient . . . had
some problem such as the loss of an insurance number
then the whole admitting process could be held up indefinitely.

One of the major impacts of computerization was in patient
admitting, which was changed to the computer in 1973. There was
a significant impact on procedures. The director of admitting
attributed the impetus for this change to Wright, although the idea
was also being implemented in other hospitals in the community.
One of the main impacts of the computerized admissions system
was the ability to generate better reports, thus improving control.
According to the director of the admitting department:

When I first came here, all the reports, including the
patient census, were compiled by hand. Now all we
have to do is punch in the data on the Telex and the
following morning we have a computer printout that
has all the information that we need to generate practically any type of report. One of the main changes
that the new computerized system has brought about is
the fact that we can generate practically any type of
report that any department in the hospital wants with
exceptional speed and accuracy. . . .

However, the director also found that departments did not need all
the reports they requested:

Therefore, I followed a policy of cutting back on reports
and if the departments didn't ask for a report, I didn't
give it to them. I've been successful in cutting down
our administrative reporting to other departments, including administration. However, when I tried this
little trick on them it just didn't work. For whatever
reason, administration seems to always know what kind
of report they want.

CHANGE PATTERNS IN NURSING

The nursing function at Victory exhibited a striking amount of
change as well as interesting patterns of behavior in planning and
implementing changes. Many of the changes reflected the concern

of nurses not only for the quality of patient care but also for the improvement of nursing techniques and administrative practice in the department. The change processes also reflected the need to cope with environmental uncertainty, and one of the primary ways of coping was to keep in line with changes in the nursing profession at large.

The vice president of nursing, Ella Winters, came to Victory in 1965, eight years prior to this study, from a teaching position in her state's first LPN training school. Prior to that, she had taught nursing at a local junior college. She credits her teaching experience as the source of much of her creative thinking and many of the ideas she has instituted at Victory. She was also a frequent participant in professional meetings around the nation and in her state, and an avid reader of books and journals on management, organization, public affairs, and nursing.

Winters presented a troublesome paradox: she talked good management practice, but subordinates were often resentful and uncooperative. One nurse, for example, reported that "her main problem is that she is so insecure that she won't let competent people assist her." Subordinates also feared her extensive reading because "every time she reads a book she tries to make us do some crazy new thing we don't really need to do."

Nevertheless, Winters was a hard, diligent worker with high professional standards and carefully selected goals; she was an active agent for change. Under her leadership, nursing was one of the first departments to adopt what she called a management by objectives system, with time budgets and goal planning by her staff members. She used the goals as standards against which to compare results, following which the lists of goals were periodically revised.

However, Winters was ambivalent about her administrative role, seeing it in conflict with the clinical responsibilities of nursing:

> One of the big problems I think about a lot is whether nursing should be administrative or clinical. I don't know which is right. We have changed from being clinical to being very administrative. A director of nursing can't be clinical but she must be very close to the clinical side of things. She has to know the clinical side.

Winters reported that she disliked the changes in her work that resulted from increasingly complex administration. In 1970, her title was changed from director of nursing to vice president of nursing. Asked what the effects of this change were, she replied that:

> I attend a lot of meetings I didn't have to go to before.
> Most of my time is involved with the people higher up.
> I meet once a week with all the vice presidents. I
> meet with the joint council of physicians and trustees
> quarterly, that's for the whole Norfield complex. I
> don't go to the executive committee meetings of physi-
> cians, but the other vice presidents do. I don't really
> care. I don't want to go to those meetings. I accom-
> plished a lot more when I was director of nursing than
> before I got so involved with the bureaucracy. It frus-
> trates me when I'm not able to do the job I ought to do
> for nursing care. This is why I don't think we can go the
> administrative route.

Winters was also somewhat ambivalent in her attitudes toward change. The following comment shows her awareness of uncon- scious, gradual change and the impact of imposed change. It also reveals a certain apathy toward changes having their sources out- side the profession of nursing:

> So many changes we undergo are actually unconscious
> changes. They're not always planned. For example,
> computers. We just take them in our stride. It's
> kind of an imposed change. Things come about and
> we all acknowledge their existence. One problem is
> that with so much imposed change going on, it makes
> it hard for us to undergo deliberate or planned change.
> Enthusiasm is needed, but people who are already
> tired of changes they have to go through are more
> likely to say no than to be fired up over it.

Three sets of innovations were nevertheless of far-reaching significance for the nursing department. The first was the estab- lishment of a system of unit coordinators. The second was a change from primary nursing care to team nursing. The third was the creation of several nurse specialist positions in Winters's office. Let us consider each of these in turn.

Unit coordinator positions were established at the time the linking-pin structure was devised. The unit coordinators are di- rectly responsible for 24-hour-a-day coverage of nursing services within their assigned units. They direct the nursing staffs on all three shifts but they themselves work only the day shift. The chief benefit was described as achieving flexibility of nursing assignments during emergency situations. Pressure for this change originated in the external environment, as a trend in the nursing profession. According to one of the evening supervisors:

It seems to be a trend . . . in some hospitals. It also
seems to work better in some situations than others.
One of the main benefits is in an emergency where
nurses are needed immediately and this system seems
to be able to move personnel around very well. However, the specialty units such as intensive care are
pretty good at covering their units themselves.

The duties of unit coordinators vary according to the types of
cases on each floor. One of them provided the following basic description of her duties:

I have the indirect or overall responsibility for patient
care 24 hours a day. I have to make sure that there is
a balance of coverage. I am responsible also for the
management of all the personnel on all three of the
shifts. If an employee has a problem, it is my responsibility to have a conference with that employee and
tell her what the problems are as I see them. I evaluate subordinates on either a six-month or annual basis.
Supervisors who are really gung-ho will do it every six
months or possibly oftener. . . . I feel that employees
are not evaluated enough in most nursing units. Another of my responsibilities is to make sure the unit
stays within its budget and that it is supplied with the
necessary equipment. . . . It is also one of my duties
to work closely with staff education in planning in-
service programs for the employees. This duty over-
laps with another of my responsibilities, which is to
orient new personnel, with the help of staff education.
Another basic duty is disciplining and firing employees.
I don't do the actual hiring and firing, but I have a lot
of influence on the individuals who do. Another of my
primary duties is to function as administrative liaison
between the nursing officials and the hospital and my
employees. Therefore, I have periodic meetings to
keep the employees informed. I can do this any way I
choose as long as I communicate with them, but I prefer
to meet with them personally to let them know what's
happening and to air their feelings on things that are
happening within the hospital.

With such responsibilities as these, unit coordinators have
ample scope for creative tasks. One such unit coordinator was described by an evening supervisor as follows:

> In the surgical intensive care unit I have a person who
> I think is one of my most innovative and creative unit
> coordinators. Recently she suggested that we modify
> our nurses' problem-oriented medical record, not the
> system that you are probably familiar with but one that
> uses a color coding which would be a blue for day, red
> for afternoon, and green for night. She and I both agree
> that this system is more likely to make the nursing care
> plan more efficient and effective administratively. She
> has also implemented lately what we call a pre-op orien-
> tation. This learning experience is for patients who are
> going into the surgical intensive care unit [SICU]. The
> nurses from SICU talk with patients and tell them what to
> expect . . . they tell them how to cough and how to
> breathe, and so forth, so that when they wake up after
> surgery in SICU they can help us more, and I think the
> net result is less apprehension. . . . This coordinator
> also has a unique approach to employee development.
> She puts one nurse in charge for two months at a time for
> in-service education. Therefore, it makes this individ-
> ual much more aware and sensitive to the problems in
> this area and helps to make them, we feel, a better em-
> ployee. Now our cardiac intensive care unit is new and
> our supervisor is really just getting it off the ground.
> But we are trying something new there, too—a monitor-
> ing technician. . . .

Mrs. Winters regarded the unit coordinators as a more important source of innovative action than the assistant directors on her
immediate staff:

> The way I see it, I came into this job for a change from
> the days when I was a professor. After several years
> in this position, I feel that I'm about to learn how change
> takes place. It's not at the assistant director level, it's
> at the unit coordinator's level. Some of my unit coordi-
> nators are real balls of fire.

TEAM NURSING

The second major innovative change in nursing was the establishment of a team nursing system instead of a primary nursing care
plan. In primary nursing, each RN is assigned her own patients for
whose total nursing care she is responsible. Under the team concept,

there is one team leader nurse in each of the four wings on each
patient care floor, plus one desk nurse on each floor. Each team
of nurses is responsible to the unit coordinator. Team leaders are
nurses with leadership and administrative responsibilities. At the
time of this study, the team concept had been installed, but the vice
president of nursing disliked it. She gave the rationale for the team
leader concept as one of providing patients with more services from
higher trained nursing personnel and less from nursing assistants:

> Winters: Here, let me draw you a sketch. You see,
> the hospital is in four wings that come together in
> the center like this. The main nursing station is in
> the middle. Now, under the team system it takes
> four nurses as team leaders, one for each wing, four
> RNs all tied up doing nothing but administration. It
> takes an additional desk nurse in the center. So
> that's five RNs all tied down, not doing any nursing
> really. That's what I mean by administrative rather
> than clinical. The result is that patient care gets in
> the hands of lower qualified people. They'll tell you
> if you ask them that they're doing most of the real
> nursing work.
>
> Interviewer: Aren't the duties between LPNs and RNs
> very clear?
>
> Winters: Oh, yes. Certainly. They are both licensed
> for certain permitted activities. They can both do
> things the assistant can't do. They know they'll get
> in trouble for not doing the right thing or for doing
> the wrong thing. Our nursing assistants do what
> would be ordinarily done in the home, giving baths,
> etc. But if you ask who does the real nursing, the
> nursing assistants will say, "We are."

The team nursing concept encountered difficulties because of
the more elusive nature of the changes in responsibility and accountability patterns not diffused among team members. According to
one of the unit coordinators:

> The team leader and her assistants have total respon-
> sibility for patient care for all patients in their wing.
> However, I am directly responsible for patient care
> and therefore there is no accountability by the people
> who are actually ministering to the patient directly.
> With primary nursing, responsibility for total patient
> care is assigned to each nurse in the form of a five- or

six-patient assignment. Under primary nursing, the
RN or the LPN wouldn't be allowed to delegate any
nursing responsibility to anyone else. Therefore, she
would be directly accountable for comprehensive patient care. Not only would there be the advantage of
accountability for the nursing professional but there
would be advantages to the patient. For example, the
patient would know who was individually responsible
for his care, and this tends to relieve apprehension.
Also, doctors would know which nurse was responsible. . . . Another advantage is that this type of
care would place the nurse professional at the bedside
where she wants to be.

An experiment with a change to primary nursing was initiated
at the suggestion of Winters. She favored the primary nursing concept and disliked the team nursing system, but she wanted a study
to demonstrate the value of changing back to the old system. According to Winters, the change to primary nursing would help to reverse
the trend toward more administrative and less clinical work by RNs:

Interviewer: The RNs are becoming less clinically
oriented and more administratively oriented?
Winters: That seems to be the trend. However, we
can still be within the law and experiment some.
Right now we are thinking that if patients are divided
according to degree of illness we can get the RNs
away from the administrative tasks involved in nursing practice and back to working more with the patients. This concept is called primary nursing. I
got the idea from a book I read recently entitled
Primary Nursing—A Model for Individual Care.
After reading the book, I suggested that a few of the
unit coordinators and nursing supervisors read it.
They became very interested in the concept and
therefore we formed an ad hoc committee which was
composed of individuals who were interested in it.
I believe that we are really going to do something
with it. It's a real interesting change and has a lot
of far-reaching implications, financially and otherwise, for hospitals.

Accordingly, Winters readily approved the study proposal. The
groups on the fifth and eleventh floors asked for permission to make
the study after team nursing had been in effect for over a year.
According to one of the assistant directors of nursing:

We want to see if primary nursing will be better received than our present system. We have written a
proposal for a grant to get funds to try to implement
this system. It has been tried in California hospitals
and to my knowledge it has worked fairly well except
on nights. . . . Primary nursing would do away with
the typical patient complaint of not seeing a nurse the
whole time he is in the hospital. It is oriented towards
patient education. The nurses seem to really want it.
I was rereading the goals of the nursing staff this morning and most of them say they want better patient care
and they want more time at the bedside.

And, according to a unit coordinator on the eleventh floor:

With our team approach to nursing we are structurally
divided on this floor into three wings. There is no real
personal responsibility to the RN and she will delegate
it on down the line to the LPN and nobody is responsible
in that case. Therefore we've tried to approach the
problem in terms of accountability and who is responsible. We decided that first of all we must divide up
equally among the available nursing professionals and
assign personal responsibility for keeping track of the
nursing care plan. . . . Our basic assumption has been
that when people know what's expected and who they are
responsible for taking care of and accountable for they
will not only do a better job but they will have a better
attitude when they do it. The mix of personnel that we
presently have on the teams consists of a registered
nurse, an LPN, and the nursing assistants. They are
all responsible for different segments of patient care,
and we feel that this fractionated type of care has given
rise to the standard complaint of most patients that they
didn't see a nurse professional the whole time they were
in the hospital. Patients' complaints notwithstanding,
however, we feel that the mix should consist of more
registered nurses and LPNs with less nursing assistants.
In the not too distant future nurses will see the elimina-
tion of the nursing assistant. If we can free the RN from
her administrative tasks and give her more time to spend
at the patient's side there will be more time spent on home
care and planning pre-op teaching.

The team nursing concept, by diffusing accountability and responsibility among team members, represented an erosion of the

professionalism and an increase in the uncertainty of the task environment. According to the propositions being analyzed in this chapter, this should result in a degree of innovation and increase the pressure of change. This indeed is what did occur. Not only did change pressure arise to restore the former system but protective mechanisms were brought forth to help reduce uncertainty. According to a unit coordinator, having the nursing team leader keep her own nurse's notes improved the system:

> Heretofore, the nurse's notes have been located with the patient's chart. Oftentimes when the chart is off the floor, the nurse has a lot of difficulty in signing out. What we've done is to take the nurse's notes out of each patient's chart and put them in a binder so that the team leader can be very flexible as to where she writes her nurse's notes. At the end of each shift or the beginning of each shift, these nurse's notes will be put onto the patient's chart. The end result will be to improve the accuracy of the notebooks and reduce duplication. This will also facilitate more documentation of our patient education and so there are many plusses as far as this nurse's notebook is concerned.

SPECIALIZED NURSING STAFF

The third area of nursing change consisted of a number of organizational innovations related to an expansion of nursing services to patients and beyond patients to their families. Five new nurse specialist positions were established. Four of them were described by the assistant director of nursing:

> I think the climate of change is really good. For example, in nursing, we have started some major things that no other hospital has. We now have a special nurse for pre-admissions. The doctors can call in the information and the pre-admissions nurse gets it all together. We also have an interostomal therapist. She is not an RN, but she helps patients with special problems. Another change was that we established a discharge planning nurse. She works with people who are going home, works with their families, works with nursing homes they may be entering, etc. . . . Another new type of nurse we have is a clinical specialist. She works with cardiac patients and their families, helping their adjustment processes and so on.

A fifth nurse specialist position, that of medication nurse, had an interesting history. It was instituted in 1971, then canceled, but in 1974 it was proposed again for trial on the fifth and sixth floors. The medications nurse is a professional nurse giving all medication, relieving other nurses from this task. The medication nurse program consisted of assigning to an RN or an LPN complete responsibility for handling and administering medications. The failure of the first program in 1971 was explained by the unit coordinator on the eleventh floor:

> What happened was that I volunteered my unit for this particular program without really finding out what they wanted to do. It worked well on days but it didn't seem to work in the evenings and at night when the medication nurse was off because no one really relished the job. I feel that it needs the support of individuals who really want to do it. Finally, the nursing staff voted to do away with the medication nurse in spite of obvious advantages. It just didn't receive the support it needed to make it really effective and worthwhile. I saw some advantages in it but most RNs just didn't want to give the medication. They seem to want to baby-sit with the medication cart which is almost ironical. Now, three years later, the idea has come up again but this time it has come up the organization instead of down, you might say. Most good ideas have anyway and I think it will probably work this time. The reason it failed last time was because there were not enough inputs from the nursing professionals.

According to the unit coordinator on the sixth floor, the new program stood a good chance of success in an expanded form:

> Interviewer: How do you get something new going?
> Unit Coordinator: If there is an idea that we want to try with regard to patient care or quality or anything regarding nursing, we ask for a special study and if it is a legitimate request, we can do it. For example, next Monday we are implementing an experimental medication nurse program on the fifth and sixth floors. . . . Currently, we do not have a medication nurse, whereas other hospitals do. . . . This program was tried on a hospital-wide basis three years ago but it was a flop. We're sure it can work now. It is a matter of having sound principles to govern the program. For example, last time this

program was attempted only RNs could be medication
nurses. However, this time we are allowing LPNs
also to be medication nurses. We feel this will be the
most practical way to approach this project. The
point of having this division of labor in the first place
is to free our professional nurses so that they can be
at the bedside more, giving direct patient care. Therefore, we will have an expert giving medication and we
will have our professionals free for other things.

In addition to the five nurse specialist positions instituted
under Mrs. Winters's leadership, she had plans for two additional
positions. She stated that:

We have a lot of long-range plans. We want to add
things that are not shown on the chart. For example,
we need a nurse for all hospital employee health problems. When we get it, it wouldn't need to be under me
and I don't care as long as we get one. Another thing
we are planning to develop is a research nurse. . . .
You know we have been helping with the nursing quality
evaluation studies, but we ought to have somebody to
keep working on research all the time.

The introduction of nurse specialists brought considerable
task uncertainty into the nursing function, because it substantially
changed the duties of nurses generally by reducing for many the
scope of their activities. One manifestation of this uncertainty was
found in the attitudes of the nursing administrators toward the problem of patient education. The assistant director of nursing felt that
a nurse specialist is needed for better patient education:

We're involved in some exciting new things. . . . With
the increasing accountability of nurses for patient education there has been a demand for individuals to teach
nurses how to be responsible for patient education.
Until about the last ten years nurses weren't really involved in patient education and they felt that the limit
of their responsibilities was from the time the patient
came into the hospital until he left and that was it.
Now . . . preventive medicine is becoming popular,
so attitudes about nursing care are changing. This
includes patient education. For example, we feel that
now a family shouldn't necessarily go out of the room
whenever a patient has to be put in a bed and because

we feel that the family and the patient should learn to
take on this responsibility for themselves, at least to
some extent, because if a patient has to go home and
is still in some type of convalescence then the patient
and the family are going to have this responsibility and
we try to teach them that. Diabetics must learn how to
take care of themselves to live as rich and useful life
as possible. Our philosophy is that what we can do here
is great but what we can get a patient to do for himself
is that much greater.

The vice president for nursing, however, felt that despite the innovation of the specialist positions, all the RNs should accept some
responsibility for patient education:

Another interesting innovation was the use of nursing
specialized personnel as an alternative to RNs assuming more of the patient teaching function. However, I
feel the best alternative is for the RNs to go ahead and
assume a teaching function, although we have had a
relatively large amount of success with specialized
personnel.

One change in the duties of nurses was welcomed by the nurses.
This was a realignment by the dietary department of methods for
serving the patients' food trays. According to the director:

We've just been talking about one of my innovations.
That is, our method for serving food to the patients.
This was one of the first systems to change when we
moved into our new building in 1966. The nurses de-
livered all the trays to the patients, but this didn't
work. So now my staff does it. The nurses viewed
the chore of delivering food trays as extra work. . . .
I can't remember where the idea came from, but nursing wholeheartedly supported it. They still do about
3 percent of the trays, for problem patients, but they
want us to take over this part also.

STRUCTURAL CHANGE

We have seen that Winters was able to introduce and maintain
changes that kept Victory's nursing up to date with professional and
technical advances and with the newer management concepts. But

we also saw that her methods were autocratic, and that subordinates saw her as unable to lead as she expected others to do. Her structuring of the administrative apparatus for nursing appeared modern, yet the nursing function was not performed to Wright's satisfaction.

In 1974, Wright removed the operating room nurses from the administrative responsibility of the nursing department, taking personal responsibility for the operating room nurses. Winters's 1974 report implied that the physicians were behind this change:

> There were both joys and sorrows. One of the joys of having all nursing under one head was that physicians were able to get problems through to the administration much faster. The sorrow consists of the failure on the part of nursing to satisfy the physicians.

Winters provided the following direct comments on this same change:

> Because of some of the unique problems involved, Mr. Wright felt it would be in the best interest of the hospital if he took direct responsibility for nursing in the operating room. As you know, hospitals are doctor-oriented and in competition for nurses, so in order to please the doctors Mr. Wright took over all the administrative functions of the OR. The consultant who is conducting the Index XII research project told Mr. Wright recently that 15 nurses in the OR was too many. In effect the overstaffing . . . has drained nursing personnel from the other units and it has lowered morale in the hospital. What in effect has happened is that they've taken a homogeneous group of individuals and have applied a differential work policy toward one segment of the group and not towards the others. For example, nursing personnel in the OR work every other week instead of every week like the nurses in the units do. Another example is the cardiac lab which is Mr. Ellis's responsibility. Recently they needed a nurse and therefore they contacted our best nurse in one of the units and proselytized her. When they moved her from the unit to the cardiac lab, she gave the reasons for leaving as (1) she was contacted by the lab director, (2) better hours, and (3) better salary. The inevitable result from this kind of thing is lower morale. I feel that all nursing should be coordinated under one head. Now that doesn't

necessarily mean that I want all the power, but I think that there should be a little more coordination in this respect.

We have now completed our review of conditions precedent to innovation and change, and have examined in this chapter the processes of planning and strategies designed to cope with uncertainties in the task environment through the mechanisms of change and innovation. We next turn to an examination of the evaluative processes shown by the model in Chapter 1 to include adoption, implementation, and training in education.

NOTE

1. Jon L. Pierce and André L. Delbecq, "Organization Structure, Individual Attitudes, and Innovation," Academy of Management Review 2 (January 1977): 32-33.

8

THE BUREAUCRATIC SIEVE:

EVALUATION, ASSESSMENT, AND ADOPTION

Traditional models of innovation processes give adoption a central role, but pay little attention to evaluation and assessment. Yet ideas that survive birth pangs, trial balloons, and experimentation often undergo serious examination before they proceed into the implementation and utilization stages. The model in Figure 1.3 separates the adoption process of the traditional model into a three-stage evaluation process which includes adoption decisions, implementation, and education. This chapter describes the evaluation and assessment activities and problems of the adoption decision. Figure 8.1 reproduces this part of the model.

At Victory, the processes of evaluation and assessment were sharply defined. Managers attempting changes were highly aware of the need to prove their case. They recognized fully that the hierarchy, someone "up there," makes the ultimate decisions and therefore governs the nature and direction of the justifications needed.

Two main types of situations with respect to evaluation and assessment will be analyzed here. First, there are major changes and innovations that affect more than one unit of the organization, or even the entire organization. Awareness of the proposed change is widespread, and the level of concern is likely to be high. Those affected may voice favorable or unfavorable opinions. They may influence, block, or support the change proposal. Such proposals thus undergo substantial scrutiny, and many in this group rise through hierarchical screening processes to the top echelon of management.

Many major changes are indeed originated by the executive vice president and his vice presidents. These may be the subject of suggestions or trial balloons for the lower echelons, but if they are costly or affect other parts of the Norfield system, they are screened by the executive committee of the central group or by the board of trustees.

FIGURE 8.1

Partial Model Showing the Evaluation, Adoption, and
Implementation Stages of the Innovation and Change Process

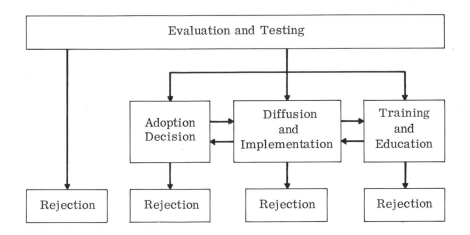

Source: Constructed by the author.

The second type consists of innovations and changes within
single units or within the work jurisdictions of particular individuals.
These are seldom noticed outside the domain concerned, except when
a person seeks credit from higher levels for some internal success,
or when the change, though localized, involves a high visibility.
Most changes in this group are relatively minor, although it is always possible for an extensive innovation or change to be confined
to a single unit or job. Many changes of this type go unrecognized
and unidentified; some may even be unconscious adjustments of individuals to the demands of their work and thus are unrecognized
by the change agents themselves. Some persons may be aware of a
change but may not perceive it as an innovation. Some are deliberately covered up to avoid possible repercussions.

MAJOR INNOVATIVE CHANGE

The principal requirements for successful change and innovation in Victory Hospital were that changes had to be logical, find
acceptance among affected people or departments, and be feasible

and cost-effective. Of these factors, that of cost-effectiveness was the most important.

Cost justifications were particularly emphasized by Wright, the chief administrator. His main standard of evaluation was the dollar. To be accepted by him, the proposed change or innovation had to undergo a careful financial analysis insofar as that was possible. Admittedly, some things were difficult to measure, especially in monetary terms:

> I think evaluation is a problem. How are you going
> to judge what innovations are worthwhile? To me the
> only test is dollars. Dollars are your common de-
> nominator. I know you sometimes can't measure but
> you have to get the best estimate.

Wright was aware that some things are more measurable than others, but he thought that everything should be measured if possible:

> An effort should be made on every front to obtain
> measurements against which comparisons can be made.
> For example, it is hard to measure the chaplain's pro-
> ductivity or usefulness. We don't know what his value
> is to the organization. Sure, they tell us that they
> counsel dying patients and their families, or they pre-
> vent suicides, et cetera, but can we measure this?
> We need to know whether they are able to reduce sui-
> cides compared to what they would be if they weren't
> working on them. In areas like this, the idea of
> measurement is not too compatible.

Just as Wright's leadership was a model for others in pressing for improvement, so, too, did his standards for evaluation apply throughout the organization. This emphasis on costs frequently led to substantial research and analysis aimed at justifying proposed changes. For example, the chief radiologist so indicated:

> Interviewer: Do you find that the administration is
>   quite receptive to suggestions and plans?
> Radiologist: Yes, we have a good reciprocity between
>   us. They are never totally negative on anything.
>   This is O.K., as long as we have some people to
>   make the studies. You see, radiology is full of
>   very expensive equipment. It takes a lot of work
>   to make any change that is going to involve high

costs. We had the same problem and went about
handling it the same way for a neurosurgery section, in a study we had to do on daily work levels.

However, innovators and seekers of change had access to resources that greatly assisted the research on which they based their
cases. In radiology, for example, plans for the new ACTA scanner
had the help of the medical records analysts:

> Interviewer: It sounds like you are involved in some
> very interesting things going on around the hospital.
> Can you tell me how innovation in one part of the
> hospital might affect your department?
> Analyst: Quite simply, I help generate the ideas.
> For example, radiology has come up with some
> new concepts in scanning devices. There's a
> piece of equipment on the market right now that
> costs $325,000, yet it's unique and does a very
> good job in what it is intended to do. Our radiol-
> ogy department felt that this equipment could
> make our department one of the leading radiology
> units in the state. Radiology, therefore, wanted
> to purchase it. The state commission, however,
> said no, because the fixed cost of this piece of
> equipment was so high and it cost too much per
> unit to pass along to the patient. . . . The guide-
> lines of the state commission are set mainly on
> the basis of the number of radiology patients
> treated. But I analyzed the data for the radiology
> department and was able to convince the state com-
> mission that in this particular specialty we did
> more than other hospitals in the community and we
> were finally granted permission to buy the equip-
> ment.

The acquisition of the new scanner, as with other medical
equipment purchased by the hospital, involved decisions by both
physicians and administrators. In Victory, the physicians decided
first, proposing the acquisition to the chief administrator. The administrator made the adoption decision based primarily on an analysis of costs, revenues, and other considerations, such as space
availability.

The CT scanner (short for computerized axial tomography)
has been used so far primarily for diagnostic brain scans, but it appears to have a potential for scans of the entire body. The British

firm EMI Ltd. had sold about 230 machines world-wide since they went into use in the United States in 1973. Pfizer, Inc. markets the ACTA scanner purchased in 1975 by Victory Hospital.

Physicians throughout the country differ in their opinions about CT scanners. Most believe it has value for brain scans, but extensive clinical evaluation will be needed before its use beyond the brain can be judged. Radiologists at Georgetown University reviewed 1,100 clinical tests, concluding that body scans were helpful but have a number of limitations, and that substantial gains in diagnostic information will have to be made to compete with standard and less expensive radiography.[1] Some physicians feel that scanners are primarily research tools and that they have not proved themselves in patient use because of their low probability of affecting the course of a patient's disease. Others claim that its value lies in improved diagnosis. Blue Cross-Blue Shield organizations have in some cases denied insurance claims for the costs of scans. Clearly, Victory's adoption of the scanning technique entailed substantial risks, including economic ones. But it typifies Victory's intention to maintain a position of leadership in the services it offers.

The scanner acquisition illustrates the enormous time burdens incumbent on professionals who seek to carry out change. The physician in charge of radiology described his role as follows:

> Interviewer: Is there a problem for you in the length of this change process?
> Radiologist: Yes, it usually results in quite a delay. For example, getting the new scanner took me five months of hard work, getting data, comparing machines. There are two main kinds we had to investigate. I estimate that I put in two to three hours a day on this project alone. I had to travel a lot to check on these machines. Then I had to write a 10- to 15-page report for my partners. We also had to go to the State Health Planning Board. You have to get their approval on anything over $100,000, and this one is going to cost $400,000. We had to study the ability of this machine to generate income so that we can amortize its cost. We also had to examine data on the estimated number of brain scans needed in the future.

The chief types of change involving significant costs relate to the purchase of new equipment and the addition of personnel. Elaborate budgetary planning was used to keep these costs under control.

Nearly all rejected changes were decided on the basis of these two criteria.

SCREENING CHANGE PROPOSALS

An elaborate decision process prevailed at Victory by which new ideas and proposals originating at lower levels moved upward until they attained the necessary higher approval. This process corresponded to the hierarchical organization pattern. Thus, change agents had to view their proposals in light of their potential treatment in the hierarchy. The chief radiological technician indicated the importance of knowing the decision makers higher up:

> Interviewer: It does help you take your ideas up to the next level?
>
> Chief: Yes, but a lot depends on who the individual is up there. For example, under Mr. Wright's policies, I can decide to spend anything up to $500, but anything more than that has to be approved by all channels—vice president, administrator, central office, and board of trustees.
>
> Interviewer: Do you feel the system is adequate for making changes?
>
> Chief: Yes, I think we have a good system. When I have a plan going, I submit it to anyone who might want to criticize it or who will be affected by it. After we take their ideas into account, the plan or proposal goes to the executive committee and then to the board of trustees for final approval.

The hierarchical screening system, as indicated by the above comments, functions as a control system for changes costing more than $500. Beyond this point, careful scrutiny prevailed. Thus, the hierarchy preserved for itself a substantial degree of power over changes.

The change process is similar for nonequipment innovations. For example, when the new call line was set up for employees to telephone their questions and complaints into a central reception unit for action, the system applied to the entire Norfield organization; thus, it had to be approved by the administrators of Victory and Bright and then by the administrative and executive committee, Manton, and the board of trustees.

The process of achieving affirmative decisions on changes that are screened by all channels was considered extremely rigorous by the department heads. Coupled with the rigid budgetary controls, bureaucracy was seen as a great deterrent to needed change. For example, Ellis indicated that, although the organization was relatively open to ideas:

> People don't rush to call ideas bad or stupid. However, payback to the organization is important. If we are unsure, then the matter has to be studied pretty hard. However, we are not compelled to rush and work and get a lot of ideas put in without upper-level approval.

Though the progress of an idea from conceptualization to ultimate fruition is difficult, it is not so difficult as to preclude discussion, analysis, and consideration. According to Ellis:

> Ideas are welcomed here at Victory and we get a lot of them. But the way along is hard. The process through the organization is not easy, and the sponsor of an idea does not find it easy to make progress. However, we encourage working on ideas. For example, if I had an idea for some kind of home-care plan or day-care nursery system around here, Bill Wright would let me go ahead and work on it even if he was biased against it. I think it's because something might come of it. He might find a diamond in the rough.

Strong budgetary controls exercised by administrative officers appeared to intensify conflicts with members of the medical staff. Physicians, particularly those associated with laboratories, feel intensely their needs for new equipment, but such changes can be blocked by the unassailable posture that "we don't have the money now." Resentment of budgetary problems preventing change was typified by comments of the director of the pathology laboratory:

> Interviewer: What about the traditional alleged conflict between the medical staff and administrators?
> Director: Well, I think it's better than people think it is. It's really an exaggeration to think of it as a constant conflict. When I first came here I thought we didn't have any at all. However, I'll have to say that now we do have some conflict.
> Interviewer: What would be an example?

Director: Well, most of it revolves around money.
Equipment, for example. As lab director, I think
I ought to have a say in equipment expenditures,
and they don't let me have any part of it. It really
makes us mad. I'm not actually frothing at the
mouth because there's no use jumping up and down
yelling all the time, but I don't think it's right to
have equipment and building decisions made when
we need things in the lab and don't have a chance
to indicate that. For example, the administration
built a fancy new building to keep supplies in. We
didn't need that fancy building and we didn't have
anything to say about it. I'm sure that it cost us
some new equipment we ought to have here in the
lab.

Interviewer: So, if new buildings go up, you wonder
whether it is coming out of your needs?

Director: Yes, that's about it.

Interviewer: Do you feel this way about the new intensive care unit buildings that are going to be
going up?

Director: Well, no, that's different. Patient care
is involved there and we need to do the things that
will improve patient care. But we didn't need
that fancy building to take care of our supplies.

THE PERSUASION PROCESS

Several strategies were designed to advance an idea along its
way toward implementation and utilization. Overcoming budgetary
and cost hurdles through study and analysis was only the beginning.
The proponent of a change usually had, in addition, the problem of
finding a strategy of persuasion directed at getting the cooperation
of others or heading off their opposition. Thus, persuasion is related to the implementation processes described in the following
chapter.

The strategies most frequently observed included selling the
idea to the executive vice president or the vice presidents, participation of subordinates or others affected in planning stages, the use
of outside consultants, and co-optation. All these involved person-
to-person relationships, relying heavily on the interpersonal skills
of people.

An example of the participative strategy of persuasion is provided by the comment of Vice President Ben Watson:

Interviewer: Would a new idea go over here if you
brought it in? How does your organization get
going on new ideas?

Watson: If I get fired up over something, I get into
a conference with my department heads who would
be concerned with it. I always want to involve all
the people. We study the problem very carefully,
especially with long-term employees, who are
typical here at Victory. We like to use participative decision-making methods to get all the facts
we can before we go ahead.

Selling an idea to subordinates or other affected persons by
itself is usually not enough. Since the evaluation process follows
hierarchical structures, all levels are targets for persuasion and
justification. Therefore, if someone in the top echelon is sponsor-
ing an idea, the administrator wants to know the reactions of those
below. A useful strategy is to display enthusiasm along with a willingness to accept reactions from those below. If an idea originates
further down, at departmental levels, the best strategy beyond economic justification is to demonstrate enthusiastic grass-roots support and thus co-opt the higher managers. This kind of comprehensive view of the persuasion process was indicated by Ellis, who had
to sell changes to Wright as well as to his department heads:

Ellis: I think people, most of us anyhow, are interested in change. But change is hard to get on a
one-to-one basis, especially if there are conflicting objectives, lack of time, et cetera. I've been
talking about innovation mainly from the bottom up.

Interviewer: How about from the top down?

Ellis: I'll give you an example. I discussed with Bill
Wright a while ago an idea about the feasibility of
developing an outpatient clinic, maybe some kind
of building, maybe a storefront operation downtown
or whatever. On something like this, he would say
that he has to have the feeling that it will fit into
our operations generally and that it will harmonize
with the rest of our activities, plus we need the inputs from the other people who are going to be affected and assuming that funding policies, such as
whether we accept federal grants or not, can be
worked out. He does not delegate stuff like this,
but if a guy wants to do his thing he ought to be
able to try it, if he can sell it.

Great care was used by Wright whenever a change was mandated from the central office—a type of change that in many organizations would be instituted by fiat and accepted without the effort to persuade. An example is provided by the way in which the new position of vice president of business administration was created. The idea originated with Hayfield, the financial officer for the Norfield complex. He wanted a counterpart in Victory who would enhance liaison and intercommunication. He asked Wright to establish and staff a position. However, the vice president who was hired for this job indicated Wright's perceptiveness in properly paving the way for change, even though he did not allow the matter to be delayed by extensive discussion at lower levels:

> Interviewer: When a new change or program is raised, does it create any stirring or excitement among people? Do people talk about it and react to it?
> Nelling: It depends on how it is sold. Mr. Wright realized, for example, that creating my department would put someone in who would be meddling in other affairs. Even if this is done with a good spirit, it is well to be cautious. In such a case a good selling job is a great help. Mr. Wright did an awfully good job of advanced selling before the job was actually established. So much goes on around here that people's don't have time to hang around the water cooler and talk about everything. With a lot of things going on, they don't get a chance to pay too much attention to any one thing.

Many areas of change in a hospital involve persuading physicians to accept the changes even to the extent of modifying their own practices. For example, the staff of the nursery came up with a plan for prenatal classes for prospective parents, including allowing fathers to attend and to observe the birth of their child, with the doctor's permission. According to the nurse in charge of special projects, resistance decreased over time as the project gained experience, overcoming reservations of both doctors and nurses:

> Of course, this new approach is not unique at Victory. It is gaining popularity throughout the nation, but it is new to our organization and we had to go through the steps of gaining acceptance from doctors and from certain individuals who were working in the labor and delivery and nursery areas. Most of the doctors have come around, but some still don't like the idea and

they are allowed to permit or deny the father being in
the delivery room. It was a very definite change and
we still have some resistance from the nursery
nurses. I should say that there is less resistance
now than there was in the beginning primarily because they've been able to see that the positive things
about the idea outweigh the bad things and it allows
the nurse to have a broader perspective than just her
nursery or her delivery room.

In pushing for another change, the head of the cardiovascular
laboratory had to focus on persuading and co-opting physicians:

One day my people and myself, in line with the objectives of our unit, were looking at one of the big kill-
ers here in the hospital, pulmonary embolisms, and
wondering what we could do to decrease the number
of fatalities resulting from this condition. . . . We
found that IPGs were a solution to this phlebitis and
we asked for $1,750, which we got immediately, to
buy equipment. As a result, the death rate from this
particular condition has been cut 50 percent. We are
not taking full credit because we only had the equipment and pushed to have doctors become more aware
of the problem and test more often. So a lot of success was the result of the increased attention that
the doctors gave this condition. I'd like to see more
done in this area. However, Victory is a clinical
hospital. We don't do any research here. I'd like
to see a research hospital take this IPG and see if
it can even be improved on.

Another example of persuasion for change shows how sanc-
tion or endorsement from Wright alone was not enough, but that
persuasion of nurses and medical staff members was necessary.
This change involved abandoning the policy of contracting out maintenance and repair services for biomedical equipment and machinery and replacing it with an in-house maintenance group. This was
an idea of the director of maintenance, who saw his plan as evolving
from studying cost problems and listening to technicians who came
in under contracts. His strategy was to get permission for a modest beginning and nurture the idea's growth over time:

. . . It was my idea, but it was the culmination of
observation of technicians and the cost involved in

the service. After watching these maintenance technicians for a number of years, I realized that much
of the maintenance they perform was really superfi-
cial and not very complicated. With the proper tools,
I felt that I or maybe someone else could train technicians to do this type of work in a hospital. It
wasn't easy, however, to sell Mr. Ellis on the idea,
but I was persistent and after a time was successful.
He let us try a few instruments, and as we achieved
success, the idea seemed more and more practical.
I've gotten wholehearted support and soon I'm sure
we will be doing even more in this area.

Ellis's account squares with that of the director of maintenance, but provides further illumination:

Interviewer: Could you tell me more about what's
in this biomedical maintenance program?
Ellis: Servicing this equipment is an interface job,
a confidence game, if you will. It's what people
believe, what they think is good or bad. That's
the way we sell it. We got the general endorsement of Mr. Wright on the project, but we had a
harder time selling the nurses and the general
staff. We were able to save about $10,000 a year
by doing it ourselves instead of contracting out
these maintenance services. Of course, we had
to train people to do the work.
Interviewer: What resistances did this plan encounter?
Ellis: Well, we had to get people to believe in it and
to show its good points. What interfered with this
was that we've had a habit around here for a long
time of relying on vendors. You buy some fancy
equipment, the vendor brings it in, and on the way
out of town he stops at the nearest service organization and tells them to come out and take care of
it. That way we don't know what we're getting.
We had to overcome this habit of relying on vendors.
There is still some reluctance, but we've come a
long way from the original problem.
Interviewer: And the maintenance engineer thought
up the idea?
Ellis: I have to be real candid about that. I can't
take any of the credit for the idea. At first I

wasn't sure it would work. I don't have the competencies, of course, to make a lot of the judgments.
Biomedical is only one of the department's activities and he was only one man, spread pretty thin.
He went about it by finally convincing me he had
the cooperation of one of the intensive care units
and that he had found a man to help him get the
project under way. My only concern was to bug
them to be careful and accurate, and I'll have to
admit there were times during all this when I was
worried about the outcome.

Most of the persuasion observed among managers and technicians at Victory appeared to be straightforward, devoid of devious-
ness and trickery. Bargaining, however, was widely evident, as in
the case of the pre-employment negotiations of the newly hired
director of the cardiovascular laboratory. The strategy involved
focusing on derivative benefits adding to the persuasion process.
For example, in changing to the patient profile system of dispensing
medicines, nurses wanted the pharmacy to be open on a 24-hour-a-
day basis. According to the chief pharmacist:

Before we implemented the profile system we had the
Brewer system, consisting of vending machines
available to the nurses on each floor. The nurse
would remove the drug after interpreting the medication orders from the doctor's medication request by
punching a coded card into the machine. The pharmacy of course was responsible for keeping the
Brewer machines stocked. One of the primary advantages of the Brewer system was that each floor
had a supply of drugs that was readily available and
convenient. Whenever the Brewer machines ran out,
and this happened occasionally, the night supervisor
from each floor could come down to the pharmacy
and open it with a key and remove the drugs that she
needed. Needless to say, the supervisors didn't like
this responsibility. Sometimes, this meant that the
night supervisor would have to come from home or
give the key to someone at work and have her remove
the drugs because she was responsible even when she
was off. As I saw it, the big problem with the system was that there was not enough interaction between
the nursing staff and the pharmacy. Since the nurse
had the responsibility of interpreting the doctor's

medication request, we were never quite sure if the
nurse was making the correct interpretation. We
knew that we were putting the correct drugs in the
machine; however, we weren't sure that the nurses
were able to decipher the difference between digi-
oxygen and digitoxen. . . . I felt . . . that we
needed to get rid of this Brewer system because I
didn't think it was effective, so I tried to sell an
idea of filling orders from the pharmacy and keeping it open 24 hours a day. As a matter of fact,
keeping the pharmacy open 24 hours a day was the
only way I could sell the idea to the nurses. After
the problems had been pointed out and my alternatives were generally accepted, administration assigned me an industrial engineer and we went to
work making the flowcharts and designing a patient
profile case. When we finally implemented the system, it was a real morale booster for the nurses
and administration liked it also.

Consultants play a role in the persuasion process. Often this
is a type of co-optive strategy: involve a consultant in the preliminary problem-solving planning and studies, steer the consultant to
a solution the change agent wants, then use the consultant's recommendations to bolster the case—we should do it because the consultant said we should. The pitfalls of this strategy were described
by Ellis, himself a former successful consultant, noting first the
higher failure rate of consultant's recommendations:

Interviewer: What do you mean by failure? This
    could be something suggested and tried that
    failed, or something that was expected and
    didn't come out of the consultation.
Ellis: It could be either of those two things and it
    could be a third thing, that sometimes the con-
    sultant doesn't even answer the question He
    gives you a report that's nice and neat and full
    of things interesting to him but his perception
    of our problem is mismatched, so the effort
    doesn't bring any real payoff. The manager
    using the consultant should tell the consultant
    what his expectations are and indicate the real
    nature of the problems to him. The consultant
    can't work in a vacuum.

Interviewer: Do consultants have to sell or persuade you to accept their ideas after they've done all the work?

Ellis: I was a consultant myself for a long time and I have a feeling for some of these things. I guess the consultant does have to sell. It depends on the type of consultant and the nature of the problem. Most of them write up a report which justifies their ideas. There is more sweat in doing that than in trying to sell the ideas. You see, the consultant is very ego involved. He puts so much of himself into it, he's likely to say here it is, take it or leave it.

Interviewer: I see.

Ellis: After a while I learned to psyche out a client and that way I would maybe get him to accept 70 percent of the potential of my proposals. Really, what an administrator has to do is massage the consultant's recommendations to fit the environment the consultant can fully appreciate.

Interviewer: That sounds complex.

Ellis: It is complex. It's hard for the administrator to really perceive the consultant's goal, and a consultant is never in a management role, so he may not understand that either. A consultant's time is very important to him. He is used to being very independent and values his independence.

MINOR AND INTERNAL CHANGES

Earlier it was suggested that some changes are narrowly confined or localized, having little impact on other persons or groups, and therefore requiring little or no justification or persuasion. These changes are few in number, and are so much a matter of habit in the adjustment of people to their work that little attention is usually paid to them.

In the simplest case, a change agent espousing an internal change has only to persuade his immediate supervisor. For example, when the business office manager wanted to set up a training program for clerical personnel, he proceeded as follows:

Well, first of all, I planned exactly how the program was going to run and then I told Mrs. Nelling what I had in mind. I explained that it wouldn't affect departmental operations since the training would be administered to half the staff at a time. She said that if I thought the department needed the training to go ahead and implement the program. As a matter of fact, I got the director of admissions interested in the program and she sent some of her people up to view it.

The director of neurosciences indicated a similar procedure, first selling the proposed change to the physicians and technicians concerned:

Interviewer: Once you've gotten an idea from a convention or a periodical, how is it implemented in your department?
Director: First of all, our two physicians and myself will discuss the new idea. If we decide that it is something that will benefit the department and the patients, we will discuss it with the technicians. If after this discussion we feel that the idea is still a beneficial one, we implement it.

According to Ellis, the simplicity of small changes is a desirable advantage, since the bureaucracy is less likely to be involved:

Ellis: We don't really have autonomy in a lot of these matters. We have to filter ideas through the general office, and we get too much delay structuring our decisions.
Interviewer: I see.
Ellis: The way the bureaucracy works is that it takes a lot of effort to handle a great big change. This encourages us to go ahead and make all the little changes we want to because they don't create much of a stir. Most of the small things are pretty well accepted. . . . On the big changes, though, we have to figure out whether the amount of trouble it causes in the bureaucracy is worth the results we get if we make the change. The bigger the bureaucracy, the harder the change of any significant kind.

Some types of change decisions can be made on almost purely technical grounds, when their effects are largely internal to a unit, few people are affected by the change, and when there is trust in the

judgment of the department head. This was illustrated by the decision of the director of medical records to adopt an automated system of medical record indexing. After determining through studies
that this was the best system available for indexes of this type, he
adopted it.

Minor changes, internally oriented, can also be made on a
trial basis, whereas this strategy is more difficult for major changes.
On one of the nursing floors, for example, the following trial of an
idea was described by the unit coordinator:

> Recently we started what is called "walking rounds."
> When one shift goes off duty and another takes on the
> tour of duty, the charge nurse gives an oral report,
> or sometimes it is taped, about each patient on that
> unit or wing to the charge nurse coming on duty.
> With walking rounds, instead of this report being
> given in a conference room, we give it in front of
> each patient's door so that the patients hear what is
> being said about them. They can find out something
> about their care and they also know who is going to be
> responsible during the coming eight-hour interval.
> We use this method on just one wing on the eleventh
> floor right now and it seems to work better on days
> than evenings. Of course, if the patient is asleep or
> is comatose, we give the oral report outside the
> patient's door. We feel that the patient has a right
> to know which nurse is going to be responsible for
> his care and that knowing this will relieve some ap-
> prehension. We hope that this technique will lead to
> better nursing care assessment if we can get patients
> more involved, and we hope that this will lead to
> better care.

ADMINISTRATIVE REJECTION OF CHANGE

The preceding sections have presented the key criteria which
administrators use in the evaluation of ideas and suggestions for
change. A number of successful changes were illustrated and problems relating to the strategies of persuasion were analyzed. We
turn now to a consideration of the processes at work by which change
proposals are rejected before adoption or reversed in some way
after brief trials.

The outright, immediate rejection of an idea was rare at Victory. The degree of openness prevailing in the hospital's organiza-

tion and its management styles were such that almost every proposal for change appeared to receive careful attention. An idea originating at the top was seldom carried out unless there was wide support from lower levels. Significant changes originating at lower levels were generally not pursued in the absence of support from the top, and indeed could not be pursued if budgetary restrictions were invoked from the top.

One type of failure of an idea to progress to adoption had its source in the personality or capabilities of the change agent. It is clear that in addition to the substantive desirability of a proposal based on objective criteria, the fate of an idea also depended heavily on subjective criteria. Among these were such things as colleagues' or superiors' confidence in the judgment or ability of the proposer, his reputation for successful accomplishment, and a host of emotional and personal characteristics of the proposer, such as his skill in communication. For example, one informant acknowledged his own limitations in pursuing ideas:

> Interviewer: I've heard it said that true innovators, the people that come up with the ideas, are often just tolerated by the organization and not truly accepted. How do you perceive yourself as an innovator?
>
> Informant: I'm not sure I can place myself in the category of true innovators; however, I have had a lot of good ideas that I felt weren't accepted for possibly irrelevant reasons. For example, I like to talk a lot and I believe this sometimes turns people against accepting my ideas because I throw out so many of them. Another thing, I often feel like I'm not forceful enough when I make a suggestion and let myself be overridden by someone who seems more confident that his proposal or suggestion is better.

Ideas are sometimes stifled because originators are unwilling or unable to make an objective case for a definite proposal. They procrastinate or feel discouraged, or do not feel strongly enough about an idea to do the work necessary for its adoption. For example, a typist in the admitting department indicated that she had tried many times, without success, to get push-button phones installed in her department:

> I have to dial numbers several hundred times a day and literally just wear myself out from sheer

monotony. I think that I could probably be a lot more
productive if I had a push-button phone. I've never
done any kind of time study to see how much time or
money I could save; however, I feel that maybe I
should write a letter to the administration or something because I think it would be beneficial.

Throughout the Victory organization, professional groups rejected ideas for a wide number of reasons, the principal one being
unable to sell an idea to other professional groups. Nurses, for
example, often had to gain the approval of physicians for change
proposals. Pharmacists or laboratory personnel had to reckon with
nurses and physicians as well as administrative staff. For example,
the chief pharmacist related the following problem with the nurses:

I've had trouble getting the IV additive program accepted, but not by the administration. They are in
favor of it, but not the nursing staff. . . . My recom-
mendation was that the addition of medication into IV
bottles should be done here in the pharmacy. One of
the problems, however, is that nurses have historically done this and they are reluctant to give it up. Another problem is that some drugs don't mix. Of
course, nurses can tell when the drugs don't mix in
most cases because the glucose will become cloudy
or there will be precipitation of some kind. However, sometimes the nurse can't see that the drugs
have not mixed properly. Another problem is that
IV fluids are sterile and when the nurses break the
bottle open on the floor this sterility is lost and also
the sterility of the additive is lost. Finally, there's
the problem of exact measurement. We have the
facilities in the pharmacy for exact measurements,
and the nurses don't.

Sometimes in the foreclosure of an idea, a professional group
is unconscious of its rejecting influence. The proposer prejudges
the decision and does not press his case. The chief pharmacist,
for example, expected no support from physicians for his IV additive program:

Interviewer: Have you approached doctors with your
idea?
Chief Pharmacist: No, I haven't. I really don't think
doctors would be that interested. As long as the

drug is administered, the doctor is happy. He's
more interested in the end results than the means.

Department heads interviewed in this study showed an interesting tolerance for rejection and delay. This tolerance was based
on confidence in the ultimate triumph of their case based on what to
them were its obvious merits. Commenting on this, the chief
radiological technician stated that:

> Yes, change is encouraged here. Administrators
> are willing to listen and willing to make changes.
> Not that they rubber stamp everything, but if any-
> thing is reasonable, they are open-minded about it
> and if you can demonstrate a case, you'll get your
> chance. There were a lot of things that I wanted to
> try that they turned down. Later I would find out
> that most of the time they were right when they
> said no.

Delay, though often met with tolerance, was often met also
with persistence. Asked to give an example of an idea that was long
delayed, a typist in the admitting department expressed tolerance
mixed with hope:

> Right now the chief fuss is with the admitting lab in
> the back of the admitting department. New patients
> have to go back to the admitting lab in the back of
> the admitting department and give urine and blood
> specimens before they can go to their rooms. The
> line back in the lab becomes too long and some of
> the patients are uncomfortable because they are sick.
> I don't understand why we can't just send them to
> their bed and have a lab technician go to their room
> for these samples. That's what they do in the emer-
> gency room and it seems to work. Why can't it work
> when we admit anyone? I feel that something is
> going to be done about this situation soon.

The attitudes of potential change agents toward the higher administration were generally positive. The following incident in the
neurosciences laboratory illustrates this attitude of cooperation
and, in addition, recognition of and tolerance for administrative
mistakes:

Interviewer: Does administration have any input into
your decisions for implementing new ideas?

Head of Laboratory: Yes, I'd say that administration has an input into our decisions. Equipment
is expensive. However, we're usually very conservative in our requests for new equipment and
we adhere fairly closely to the standards set by
an ad hoc committee of the two societies in our
field. These standards help justify the requests
for additional programs, additional procedures,
and equipment. We get along with administration
quite well, I feel, and have never really had any
severe misunderstanding except for one time that
I can recall.

Interviewer: Could you tell me about that misunderstanding?

Head of Laboratory: Yes. It concerned the cerebral
death recordings. Years ago when the heart-lung
machine was invented, we could keep a patient
alive indefinitely. . . . Because the machine can
keep the patient's bodily functions operating when
the brain is actually dead and has stopped giving
off life signs, neurologists and other specialists
realized the need to formulate standards whereby
we could justify taking patients off the heart-lung
machine. As you are no doubt aware, this is a
very sensitive area. However, the ad hoc committee for the two societies . . . being aware of
the legal, moral, and ethical issues involved,
wrote up a set of standards and said that we would
base our decision on an EEG on a patient. . . .
As far as the incident that precipitated the disagreement was concerned . . . the department
got a request from ICU to do a cerebral death re-
cording and administration found out about it. It
was on a weekend and it was an urgent request and
therefore was diverted to administration. However,
when administration found out, Monday morning a
note was waiting for me in my office that we were
not to do cerebral death recordings. We gather,
because of the articles that have been written in
the administrative literature, that administration
was looking at it from a legal point of view. However, the doctors, the specialists in this department, were looking at this matter from the point

of view that we had no choice but to make a decision. At any rate, when administration realized
that we must make a choice in some circumstances, they relented and allowed us to do this
particular procedure.

When the administration turned down a request, a planning
strategy was frequently invoked, showing a change agent's confidence in the ultimate outcome of the contest between needs and
budgets. For example, the chief radiologist reported that getting
turned down on a request for new equipment was extremely rare,
and the request is always built into the next three-year plan.

The element of persistence in the face of rejected or delayed
change is an important strategy. But a strategy of persistence is
more feasible for counter-delay tactics than for rejection. Delay
allows administrators to say "We are still considering the matter,"
and the proponents to say "We are still working on it." An example
of persistence coupled with delay was provided by the assistant
director of nursing:

One thing we have wanted for a long time but haven't
gotten yet is an employee health nurse. This comes
up at the nursing liaison committee every two months.
So it is still under discussion and we are still working
on it but we haven't been able to get it approved yet.

Another illustration of persistence in pursuing change was
reflected in the comment of the chief pharmacist that:

I've had two or three things that have never gotten
off the ground. With Mr. Wright I try to do a soft
selling job. First I tell him the problems in pharmacy by means of memos and letters and what not,
and then I give him my plans and alternatives for
overcoming the problems and lay out a plan of action. Then I keep reminding administration of it
over and over.

The nursing department was one of the highest generators of
change proposals. The willingness to make trials and to experiment
was correspondingly high, as were failure and rejection rates. In
the 1973 annual report, the vice president of nursing stated that
"One of the strengths of our department is the willingness to try to
change even though it hardly ever sticks." In fact, trial or experimentation sometimes appeared to be a substitute strategy for

research, planning, documenting, and other efforts to argue objectively for change. For example, the 1973 annual report recounted an unsuccessful effort to reorganize the job assignments of male nursing assistants. There were very few, and the nursing staff wanted more. The problem was the maximum utilization of a scarce type of staff member. At first they tried putting them into a central pool unit and having one available on call, so that they could be more easily located and called to duty stations. However, there was undue confusion and inequalities of distribution and use, so the system had to be canceled. Each MNA was then assigned to a definite unit coordinator.

The department of nursing tried to set up a sixth floor treatment room for esophagoscopies, gastroscopies, and proctoscopies. However, the change never materialized. A study team was sent to a nearby hospital to observe a similar organization there. But, according to the 1973 report, "somewhere in the red tape this idea got lost."

The 1973 report referred to one triumph, when nursing finally succeeded in combining nursing in three OB-GYN areas under a single coordinator. The report stated that "this had been a goal for many years. The new coordinator has accomplished a gigantic task against immeasurable opposition from many OB-GYN physicians."

The administrative ploy of taking no action in proposals for change and innovation was often frustrating to change agents because it obscured the evaluation and assessment process. There was no way to tell whether or not there had been an evaluation, or some kind of negative assessment. When the administration took no action, it typically did not provide any feedback as to why. In some cases it did not respond to queries from the change agent about the progress of an idea, plan, or suggestion. For example, a member of the business staff related that:

> I suggested not long ago that we institute a training
> program to teach the billing clerks how to bill by
> the alphabet. That is, all the clerks in the office
> would be doing all the work on patients between cer-
> tain letters in the alphabet and we wouldn't have the
> division of work the way we do now, where one clerk
> does all the insurance billing and one clerk does all
> the outpatient billing and inpatient billing. . . . My
> proposal would equalize the work load and make more
> of the clerks personally accountable for their work.
> Also, complaints could be directed to whichever clerk
> handled their account. The idea was favorably dis-
> cussed, but my boss never took any action.

One of the most interesting examples of frustration due to delay and inaction on change requests was found in the pathology laboratory:

Interviewer: If you had your choice about anything you could change in your setup, what would it be?

Director: Well, look at these budget requests. If I could change something, I would change to a definite budget of my own so that I would know what I could spend. That way I could do some planning. The way it is now, I have to kick and holler and then they don't do anything. I can't plan with any confidence at all. They don't pay any attention to these budget requests that I send in.

Interviewer: Did you take this up with higher administration?

Director: Yes. I talked to Mr. Wright about it a number of times. All he says is "We don't have our own budget either." There doesn't seem to be any hope any more. It's not really his fault, it's higher up than that.

Interviewer: I see. This looks very important.

Director: You can see I addressed this memorandum to Mr. Watson. Now we shouldn't have to go to Mr. Watson over something like this. This is a request for people and equipment.

Interviewer: What happened to this?

Director: It's been two years now and we never had any reply at all. And here's another request I sent to Mr. Manton. We didn't get any change on this either. In fact I never even got an answer about this.

Interviewer: Why don't you try to go back and get an answer?

Director: I don't keep after them. I feel it would be resented. We can only go to the administration, we can't really go to the board because as I've told you we don't have anybody there at all. But our administrators feel the same frustrations we do.

In one of the few cases of clear-cut rejection of a suggested change, the decision nourished negative feelings on the part of the business office manager:

I feel that the squeaking wheel gets the grease. . . .
Administration is very responsive to the general public and will make honest attempts to overcome problems when they become aware of them. Now, as far
as being responsive to my suggestions, I think that's
a horse of a different color. We have a problem here
in the business office in handling delinquent accounts.
The system we use is mechanized into a series of
form letters to individuals that owe the hospital
money. . . . By the amount of bad debts that the hospital has and the number that we have to turn over to
lawyers I feel that this letter system is fairly ineffective. I have suggested that we personalize these letters more by making them increasingly severe, and
that we use different colored envelopes to catch their
attention. I also suggested that this method be facilitated by a printout of delinquent accounts so I could
send these letters personally. However, my suggestions
were overridden and the mechanized system was implemented.

ADOPTION

We have thus far viewed adoption as the culmination of the un-
folding of a variety of strategies designed to influence and persuade.
Viewed from the top of the hospital's hierarchy of administration,
adoption decisions are made only after reasonable and convincing evidence deriving from planning and research is provided. But planning
and research are reinforced by the strategies of originators which reflect the extent to which they are in tune with the political, social, and
administrative realities of the hospital organization and with the personal attributes of those who decide.

The strategies reviewed in this chapter include the selling of
ideas, the marshaling of factual and attitudinal support, and the element of persistence in carrying an idea through despite difficult ob-
stacles. Finally, the strategy of the tentative "experiment" or trial
gives originators a face-saving mechanism if the trial results in
rejection.

We now turn to an examination of the diffusion and implementation aspects of our model of innovation and change.

NOTE

1. <u>Wall Street Journal</u>, November 21, 1975, p. 47.

9

DIFFUSION AND IMPLEMENTATION

The fate of an idea or proposal for change was uncertain at Victory Hospital, as it is in many if not most organizations. If an idea is brought forth at all, the originator expects that it will receive a hearing and a fair evaluation. One can assume that the originator has assessed the relative risks and probabilities of success, and has considered the personal stakes and preferences that pervade the emergent idea.

Diffusion and implementation follow from the adoption decision, and there is a subsequent training and education process by which diffusion, implementation, and testing occur. This part of the model, abstracted from the overall model shown as Figure 1.3, is reproduced here as Figure 9.1. The implementation stage extends over a period of time and is blended into other surrounding processes without discrete beginning and terminal points.

It is often the case that ideas pass through higher levels and through evaluation processes, but encounter difficulty in the implementation stage. This happens for several reasons. An idea may have substantial face validity—that is, it appears logical and feasible, so that difficulties are underestimated. An enthusiastic, well-regarded proponent may succeed in persuading others that an idea is "worth a try," even in the face of reservations held by some. Judgments about the objective criteria can be in error, especially in highly technical spheres. People make mistakes. It can also happen that an idea's consequences are inadequately assessed, and that people who should have been involved and weren't later raise overt or covert opposition. The weight of higher authority may impose a change, followed by the discovery that critical factors were not considered or that opposition was insufficiently considered. Robert Maynard Hutchins once observed that his greatest mistake as president of the University of Chicago was to believe that he had won an issue when he had 51 percent of the faculty votes.

FIGURE 9.1

Model of the Implementation Process in Relation to
Adoption and Training

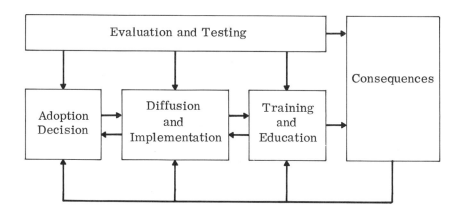

Source: Constructed by the author.

The basic posture at Victory, evident in Wright's leadership and the practices of those around him, was to base a decision for major changes on the objective elements of the case presented, putting aside subjective factors. Minor changes were often allowed experimentally with relatively less evaluation and a high propensity to reject or modify after a period of trial.

In both kinds of change, therefore, the task of implementation was a matter of continuing concern after an adoption decision was made. An adoption decision did not lead to problem-free or opposition-free implementation. Implementation itself was often a lengthy process, as much as six months or more. During this stage, unpredicted consequences had to be confronted as latent opposition became manifest or unforeseen technical problems occurred. Costs were often greater than expected and savings less.

Persuasion, study, and analysis efforts therefore had to be continuous. Changes, new programs or procedures, or new equipment have consequences that need to be monitored. Ellis, for example, indicated that his hardest work occurred after a favorable decision from Wright:

. . . When Bill Wright says sure, go ahead, I know I've got my work cut out for me. I come back to my office and really think it over before I go ahead with it. I think Bill is trying to be less of a boss and more the environment creator like the modern manager is supposed to be.

ASSESSMENT AS A CONTINUING PROCESS

Our model indicates a continuous feedback process that tempers the implementation of adopted ideas or proposals by comparing consequences to the expectations created by planning and adoption.

An assessment of advantages and disadvantages often became more detailed after a change or an innovation had been put into practice than prior to its adoption. Whereas early evaluation processes focused on possibilities for cost reduction or efficiency improvement, continuing assessment in the implementation stages permitted the consideration of more intangible, subjective values, such as human factors, as well as concrete results of the change. The adoption of a new biomedical equipment maintenance program illustrates the critical factors occurring in the implementation stage of innovation and change.

THE BIOMEDICAL MAINTENANCE PROGRAM

This new program, adopted in 1972, was highly regarded by top administrators and considered to be a success. It called for the hiring of maintenance technicians to service Victory's biomedical equipment, thereby reducing reliance on manufacturers or independent outside repairmen. Although the adoption decision was based primarily on cost savings, even this criterion became increasingly doubtful during implementation. Furthermore, unanticipated employee training and turnover problems occurred in the implementation stage.

The program came under the direction of an equipment consultant who had been involved in the planning and who was later hired on a part-time basis. Asked about the economic justifications, the consultant was ambivalent:

Interviewer: Is Victory's biomed program a success?

Consultant: If you mean, do I feel that the program is economically justified, I'm not really sure. There are a lot of economic advantages and disadvantages. . . . The problem is that a lot of the costs are intangible. One of the disadvantages is the hazard of losing people. . . . Unless you can pay people well, you will have to fight to keep the good ones in order to maintain the quality of service. . . . Where the advantages do outweigh the disadvantages . . . it is clearly worthwhile. One reason is that doctors have the say-so in what type of equipment is used, and 75 percent of the time the equipment is manufactured by companies that don't have any local service. If a company can't offer reasonable local service, nine out of ten times it's going to cost the hospital a lot in down time plus the fact that . . . the hospital has to ship the broken equipment all over the country. . . . I believe cost studies . . . would show that local maintenance outfits could often do it as cheaply as the hospital can. . . . With our biomed program, the hospital gets the advantage of economies of scale and the expertise of the personnel, but . . . there are also intangible values involved. For instance, we purchased some Honeywell heart monitors about three years ago and last year that division of Honeywell went out of business. So we had either to fix the equipment ourselves or find some other manufacturer willing to do it.

The implementation stage of the biomedical maintenance program also revealed pitfalls and difficulties that either could not be uncovered in the assessment stage of an idea, or which were ignored or given a low priority:

Interviewer: Why do you feel that the biomed program is the best alternative?

Consultant: In a hospital large enough to have this type of equipment, it is worth having a program to maintain it. I feel that it could work a lot better though. There are a lot of prima donnas in the hospital, so you will find different types of equipment doing the same type of job in different parts of the hospital. Another problem that developed

was that we don't get the service manuals. Now
I'm not saying that . . . we couldn't demand service manuals. But it doesn't work that way. . . .
The manufacturer ships the piece of equipment
direct, and engineering won't even know it's here
until six months later when the service contract
or the warranty runs out and they call on us to
fix it. . . . If maintenance is going to be responsible for equipment, we should have some input into the purchase.

Interviewer: Does lack of standardization from one
manufacturer to the next seriously affect the biomed program?

Consultant: It hinders us a lot but then, what is the
alternative? Under our economic system you
can't demand that a manufacturer make his equipment in certain ways because the only way you
could effectively do that would be through government control. . . . With the biomed program we
just try to live with such problems as the lack of
standardization and the lack of understanding between the maintenance and other departments in
the hospital. For instance, . . . I've arranged
for our personnel to watch a heart catherization
and I believe it will give them special appreciation
for jobs that are being done with the types of equipment that we service.

The implementation of the new biomedical equipment maintenance system also provides an example of the need for training
to implement change. The training, plus space and equipment repair problems, greatly extended the time required for implementation. According to the maintenance consultant:

We've been attempting to implement the system here
for about the last year. . . . The system has not
been implemented completely simply because of some
of the physical and personnel limitations that I've encountered. . . . For instance, we have to educate
our people in how to take care of this equipment and
this is a time-consuming process.

The presence of the part-time consultant who helped to originate the biomedical maintenance program reveals that in addition
to training itself, the availability of resource persons is critical in

the process of implementation. The director of maintenance explained how the program developed around the part-time consultant:

> The new program takes an awful lot of work, especially
> for in-service training. You can have a good electronics
> man, a really bright guy with a lot of potential, but
> you've still got to take the time to teach him about each
> machine, how it works, how to work on it so that he can
> get a feel for it. . . . I knew that I didn't have the
> level of technical competency to implement the system
> myself. So, when I heard an old friend of mine, Ted
> Forsgren, was retiring from a local surgical supply
> company as a maintenance man, I asked him to see
> me. I explained what we were trying to do and made
> an offer for him to come on a part-time consulting
> basis to help me implement the program. By the way,
> he's still here. He had some good ideas and aside
> from his teaching, he made some changes on his own.
> For instance, we have some good EKG machines that
> we were not using because they were old. Now the
> fifth floor has monitors that do graphic recording of
> the heart. Ted suggested that we rig up one of these
> old EKG machines with a graphic recorder and we
> could use it as a backup when one of our regular EKG
> machines went down. Heretofore we had to pay
> $1,100 to rent an EKG graphic recorder when one
> went down. It cost us only a nominal fee to rig up
> one of the old machines as a backup and so we saved
> a lot of money. As a matter of fact, one of the
> nurses told me that she preferred the old EKG
> machine rigged up with graphic recorder to the regu-
> lar machine because of the type of recorder that it
> had. . . . Ted has really been a source of inspira-
> tion around here.

Those receiving the services of the new biomedical maintenance program regarded it favorably, but they, too, alluded to problems of instability of the personnel involved. For example, the head of neurosciences indicated that:

> Prior to the implementation of the biomedical pro-
> gram I did most of the preventive maintenance work
> and a lot of the light electronic repairs. You can't
> help but learn something about electronics when you
> operate these machines. Also, the maintenance of

the equipment is enhanced by the fact that many of
the parts are interchangeable. Also, many machines
have auxiliary channels that we can use when one
channel goes out. Therefore we don't experience a
great setback when a piece of equipment goes down.
I cooperate with the biomedical program as much as
I possibly can because I can see not only a cost saving for the hospital but also a time saving. The only
problem I can see is that it's not going to work very
well unless they can stabilize their personnel. In
the last year, I have had to work with three different
people. However, because of the possibility of saving money and time I'm going to keep working with
the program, hoping that it will eventually be successful.

The new biomedical equipment maintenance system succeeded
because it had the support of top administrators, an enthusiastic
change agent who could be persuaded to direct the program, and
generally favorable attitudes on the part of users of the service.
Its difficulties centered upon staffing, turnover, and the need to
keep proving itself by making the new services better than the old,
thereby justifying the cost-benefit promises needed to secure its
adoption.

DIFFICULTIES IN IMPLEMENTATION

Even after thorough planning and careful adoption decisions,
the implementation process usually encounters difficulties. Interdepartmental relationships may not be smooth at first. Employees
must not only learn new methods, but come to accept them as a new
way of life. Such training takes time. Managers must also guard
against the tendency to slide back into old methods, or to alter procedures without reference to the basic plan. We also found that un-
expected space allocation problems resulted from adoption decisions,
and that substantial reservations about computerization continued
for some time after adoption.
One example of backsliding was found in the implementation of
the Brewer system of medication, which was adopted in 1971. This
system requires pouring medicine at the time it is to be given, but
five years later one of the nursing supervisors reported that prepouring of medications was still widely done by nurses.
Implementation was handicapped in many cases by the impact
of changes on space allocations, especially when the change consisted

of new equipment. Space scarcities, frequent remodeling, and the purchase of new and often larger pieces of equipment all led to a substantial disruption of the physical environment and feelings of difficulty and discomfort on the part of organization members. For example, the nursing education staff was frequently shifted from one location to another. At the time of this study, it was located in the adjacent Professional Office Building. According to the nursing education director, "We are a nonpaying occupant, so we get moved around a lot and this always creates a big hassle."

The chief radiologist reported that a large piece of equipment valued at $10,000 was not being used because of the cramped, inadequate space available, causing radiologists to prefer reading x-rays one at a time instead of in groups as provided by the large piece of equipment. He said that "If we could make the facilities right, we'd have a better chance of going ahead with this kind of change." The chief radiological technician, who managed the facilities, also viewed space allocation as a problem; owing to remodeling caused by the installation of a new brain wave scanner, he was about to lose most of his space for filing photographs and x-ray negatives.

The pressure on physical space as a result of acquiring the new x-ray scanner affected patients through reduced waiting room space and physicians by depriving them of office space. The scanner was very large, requiring a 40-foot by 40-foot room. In the words of the physician heading the radiology group:

> Here I am sitting in the resident's office. We are so cramped for space the doctors don't even have any offices. Several of us work in here but we are rotating with four residents. The reason is we . . . are planning to buy an ACTA scanner. We're spending about $300,000 on the basis of a gift we're getting. We are going to have to change everything around. You saw across the hall that we have already turned offices into x-ray rooms. We had to have some more room for our cobalt therapy. We are making therapy rooms out of all the office space, and even the waiting room is going to have to go. Instead of coming through the lobby the way you came in, our patients will have to come in through the therapy room door on the other side.

On a subsequent visit, the researchers found that the layout changes to accommodate the scanner had been made. New signs in the main lobby directed patients to a new and smaller waiting room.

The spacious appearance of the lobby had deteriorated, and there was increased commotion due to the changed traffic patterns of both patients and members of the hospital staff. Soon thereafter, the researcher noted that the entire main lobby of the hospital had been refurnished. There was new furniture, and new patterns of furniture arrangement. Mr. Wright reported that even a minor change such as this was disruptive:

> It seems that the amount of trouble generated by change is way out of proportion to its importance. Take that new furniture we got down in the lobby that created all kinds of pandemonium. . . . It was upsetting to everybody and it was chaos getting that job done. But it wasn't a very big item in terms of money. On the other hand, you can get a lot of expensive new equipment to be installed in the operating room and you don't have any problem. That will go very smoothly.

The optimism and enthusiasm for an innovation or change often fade when the realism of implementation is confronted. Technical difficulties often reignite the opposition of dissidents who failed to prevail against the change and have difficulty carrying out the changes. This was widespread in Victory with regard to computerization. The director of admissions, for example, indicated that:

> It doesn't even save me time because I have to do everything I used to do and more. The main way that the system has affected our department is to change the work load in the department and for the staff. That is, the staff has had to become more technically skilled in order to use the Telex and interpret the data. The work load has changed in that not only do we report things initially on certain forms but we also have to use the Telex which means that we do everything twice. Eventually, we'll have a Telex in every office and hopefully it will save time.

Similar implementation problems were indicated for the new computerized admitting system by the data control coordinator:

> The CRTs help a lot in our reporting or controlling of the output of information. This equipment has reduced our search time and given us more accurate and up-to-date information. Therefore, it has reduced the amount of time we have spent with rejections,

that is, redoing patient charges because the information was old. But controlling output is only one
phase of our operations but it is where the biggest
problems occur because we have to focus all the information for the computer when we put it in. However, when we take it out, it's only bits and pieces.
For example, the admitting department went on a
computerized system not long ago and the people
using it weren't too computer-oriented. Therefore,
we had a lot of problems in patient indexing. When
patient data is put into the system wrong, it's really
bad because the effect can be far-reaching, especially for revenue and charges. What happened was that
we had the patients indexed last names first and admitting was putting patients in by first name and then
last name and it was impossible for us to find the
patients. Naturally, I informed them of the problem
and tried to help them overcome it, which they did,
but in the meantime we were having to scrutinize
practically all of the admissions and this was taking
up a lot of our time.

The typists in the admitting department feared loss of skills
and resisted learning to use the new equipment. One indicated that
the information provided was too brief and the training was inadequate:

A Telex in every office will mean that each admitting
clerk can work directly with the computer and punch
in the data on an hour-to-hour or minute-to-minute
basis. There has been resistance to the idea because some of the typists feel that they are going to
lose their typing speed; however, the main reason is
that they just fear having to learn to work with this
machine. They believe it slows them down until they
become used to it. However, in the long run, I think
they will see that it saves everybody time because we
won't have to type the data all in at the end of the day.
What we're doing now when we admit a patient is a
duplication of work. First, we take down all the information on one sheet, then transfer it to the computer at the end of the day. It seems useless since
we could put it directly into the computer from the
moment we get it. . . . When we went from the old
system of admitting to the new automated system, we

only had a one-hour meeting on a Sunday afternoon
and a code book to tell us how to talk to the computer and that was it. The consultants gave only
one lecture to the day crews that work the regular
work week and to the weekend crews.

In the business office, too, the new computer system posed
problems. While overt resistance was not apparent, a continuing
preference for the old system lingered long after the change was
instituted. According to a financial counselor:

It's very convenient. When we started our computer
facilities in 1971, we contracted with a consulting
firm for our department to have two data display units
for our patient accounts. These display units can give
us an instantaneous status report of any patient account
we have on our books and this is very beneficial in the
disposition of accounts. Our entire accounting system
at the central computer facility is based on the IBM
SHAS program, the Shared Hospital Account System.
Although the SHAS program handles the basic functions of billing and posting fairly well, in my mind
the older ledger card system is hard to beat. If I had
had my way, I would have just automated the old ledger
card system. It consisted of a card with the patient
information on one side and the charges on the other.
The old ledger card system took longer to use than
our new computerized system. However, the logic
as far as I was concerned was a lot easier to understand. One problem with the SHAS program, for example, is that there is no way of knowing when the
deductible on an insurance policy has been paid.

The physician in charge of the pathology laboratory cited his
reservations on computerization as follows:

Everything is getting automated these days. There
are different ways to look at it. In a way, you give
a lot of additional services but not necessarily for
less money. You need about the same people. In
fact, you need a few additional, better-trained
people to take care of the stuff. But you give more.
The overall cost is not lower. Your quality control
problems are the same. Our administrative costs
at the lab are 10 percent of the total lab budget.
This seems awfully high to me. . . .

A final type of difficulty in implementation occurred when earlier cost estimates turned out after adoption to be wrong. This usually resulted in abandoning the change and returning to the former system. This happened in nursing, where one of the unit coordinators reported that:

> Another innovation that was implemented when we moved into the new hospital here was a system whereby a refrigerator was kept stocked on each nursing unit so nurses could go to the refrigerator for things such as juice and light foods. Mr. Wright felt this system would relieve a lot of administrative work on the part of the nursing staff. However, as it turned out, we had to keep two people working full time to keep the refrigerators cleaned out and stocked properly. We seemed to be defeating our own purpose. . . . We were no better off financially than when we kept all the nourishment down here in the dietary kitchen. After a time, Mr. Wright agreed with me that we should scratch this program and put the nourishment back down here.

MANAGING FOR EFFECTIVE IMPLEMENTATION

We have seen that the changes adopted by Victory's managers were usually based on economic criteria, with cost savings the major criterion. This placed a heavy burden on the implementation stage, where unanticipated difficulties, predominantly in the human sector, had to be worked out as changes progressed toward fulfillment.

Implementing new programs, procedures, or other changes is at best a costly, time-consuming process, but is an essential aspect of successful change. Commitments to make changes are usually strong, and face-saving retreats are difficult to manage. Thus pressure builds up to counteract the difficulties experienced in implementation.

In Victory Hospital, we observed several effective implementation strategies designed to make a change or innovation work out. These strategies had several things in common: they take time, they cost money, and they require the commitment of leaders who sponsor or accept the change. Among the key strategies were training, attitudinal reinforcement, and participation techniques.

There were two purposes behind training and education as observed in the Victory situation. One was to adapt technical skills to the demands of new equipment or procedures. Another was to gain philosophical or psychological acceptance by persuading those affected to end overt resistance and cooperate with changes. The former problem is a straightforward matter of technical training; the latter is a more subtle process of education leading to attitudinal change. Both processes may be necessary to implement a given change within a particular unit.

Training is costly because it takes time, and results are delayed. Training time requirements not only posed delays in the biomedical equipment maintenance and computerization changes discussed earlier but also in neurosciences, where it took nearly a year to bring a new EMG machine into use. According to the head of neurosciences, technical training was the main problem:

> It took us almost a year to make the new EMG operational. The problem was that we had to train a technicial to operate it. Therefore, we sent one of our new technicians to a three-month training course at the Mayo Clinic. Then we sent this same technician for additional training to another three-month program; therefore, it was six months before she was ready to operate the machine. Then we had to acquaint the staff with the fact that we had the machine and that using it would help them. We can't advertise the machine, so we have to do it discreetly. So it was about a year before the machine was used anywhere near capacity. One of the key factors was not only the training of the technicians but also that the doctors had to become familiar with the equipment.

A more difficult implementation problem is posed where technical or professional training alone is not sufficient. Efforts directed at attitudinal change are required. The new medication nurse program provides an illustration. The attitudinal problems were intensified by the failure of an earlier program in 1971, which had been adopted that same year by an autocratic decision of the director of nursing. It failed almost immediately because the nurses would not accept it. The new program was adopted in 1974 on a trial basis on the fifth and sixth floors, and this time the RNs were permitted to vote on whether the program would go in and how it would be set up. To further improve the chances of success, the staff education nurse was brought in. According to one of the unit coordinators:

> Starting Monday, we are going to implement the medication nursing program and this will free a lot of our

RNs and LPNs. It is going to be a big change for
them and I am fearful that they are going to be uncertain. Maybe this is the weakest part of the program right now. Tomorrow . . . the staff education
nurse is coming up here to have a talk with the employees and tell them, I'm sure, that this is their big
chance. Since the administration of medication is a
big part of the day for the nurse professional and we
are in effect wiping that out, the staff education nurse
can help us explain it to our group.

The voting process was accompanied by discussions among
the affected group members; the discussions led to ideas that
assisted in the implementation. According to the unit coordinator:

The first time this program was initiated the main
people who were pushing it were the nursing execu-
tives and I believe this is probably why it was a flop.
Currently, the people who are pushing this program
are from staff education. They came to me first and
asked me how I would like it and I told the director of
staff education that I would have to ask my people how
they felt about it. We had a meeting at which we openly discussed the pros and cons and how we could head
off any bad effects this medication program might
have. Practically everyone agreed that they wanted
it but they didn't want it like it was tried last time.
They wanted to have the LPNs as medication nurses
also. This feedback caused some changes in the way
the program was tried and I believe it is going to
work this time.

As time passes following an adoption decision, organization
members either succeed in aborting the change or through learning,
training, persuasion, or trial become acclimated to the change or
accept the inevitable. In Victory, the strategies of participation
and involvement were very effective in blunting opposition to change
and in smoothing the pitfalls of implementation.

In the preceding example from the nursing department, a voting process was utilized, and this was a common participation technique at middle and lower levels of the organization. Other participative strategies went beyond voting to include involvement in the
planning and execution stages. This process occurred in the implementation of the new computerized admitting process, for example.
According to the director:

The idea for a computerized admission program had been around for a while and people were naturally dreading its implementation. I think the basis for the resistance probably was insecurity. None of the employees had ever worked with a computer. They were all used to typewriters and not Telexes. Everyone was scared because of all the learning they knew that they were going to have to go through, such as how to code, make inputs, and stuff like that. However, we worked around the clock to make sure the department was ready before we tried to implement the system. The idea was to get the employees involved in implementing the system and make them feel like they were part of it. I knew that if they learned enough they would become confident of their ability to run the new system and therefore we'd be successful.

Participation and the improvement of internal communications were also important in implementing the new computerized admitting procedures, according to the director of admissions:

I felt that participation was not only helpful in implementing that program but also in changing the whole attitude and focus of the department. I had just been promoted to department head, and my old boss had told me that a participative approach wouldn't work. Her idea of supervision was the old iron hand and velvet glove approach. My ideas are different. I feel that we have good relationships here in the department now. I like people to feel that they are a part of the department and I like them to have all available information. The old supervisor had a habit of not communicating with all the employees. She would confide in only a few and this I feel was bad for morale. Therefore, I communicate . . . all the information I get from administration, barring anything that is confidential. I believe that it takes everyone working together to make a good department and one of the main ways to accomplish this unity is by good communications. When the department implemented the computerized program system we actually had the day shift coming in at 2 a.m. in the morning practicing on the new equipment and working with the new system. We had a deadline of six weeks and by

a concerted effort we were able to implement the
new system when we were still supposed to be
running a dual system for a few days.

The importance of participation as a requirement for successful change was reinforced by a comment of one of the management
interns attached to Wright's office:

No innovation can be forced. It has to be voluntary
to some extent. It also depends on the issue. Let's
take an example. Say the chief administrator has a
great idea and he goes down to dietary and he starts
telling people what to do to implement his idea. Unless those people have participated in the development
of the idea or are prepared for the change, chances
are the administrator's innovation is going to fail.

When a laboratory or other technical unit adds new equipment,
close liaison with physicians is needed. Implementation thus depends on the participation of physicians in planning the purchase of
new equipment, in encouraging them in its use, and in assisting
them in learning about it. This is illustrated by the following comments by the director of inhalation therapy:

Interviewer: Do you play a role in the physicians'
education about new ideas and techniques in the
field of inhalation therapy?
Director: Yes, we do, because most physicians
don't have time to read all the medical literature
and they need information from outside sources.
Therefore, physicians who are not specialists
. . . are very interested in most new ideas that
I mention to them. For instance, not long ago
there was a new device available for the volume
ventilator. It would help the patient adjust to not
being on the respirator. I mentioned it to the doctor to see if he would use it before I bought the
equipment. I'm certainly not going to buy equipment that the physicians won't let me use. Therefore, I get the physicians' inputs into our purchasing decisions. You would never see these relationships on the organization charts of a hospital. Although it's not readily apparent, in this type of
hospital physicians can and do make changes and
the administration wants to make sure that their
needs are met.

In sum, the proponents of changes, particularly innovative ones, are not free of responsibilities after their ideas are adopted. The implementation stage brings the need for training and educational efforts which, if not well thought through, can result in the reversal or abandonment of the change. Strategic planning and the involvement of group members are therefore required for implementation by refinement and adjustment. Thus, there is a need for further analysis of change agent roles and behavior as changes exert their effects over time. The chapter following is devoted to this problem.

10

MANAGERIAL ROLES AND
CHANGE AGENT BEHAVIOR

The view of innovation and change presented in the model we have been examining is one of sequential and simultaneous processes which occur in the organizational framework of the hospital. These processes occur insofar as change agents utilize them as the system in which they operate and through which they can manipulate its constituent opportunities. Thus, a strategic element in innovation and change is the use of organizational or social roles by which individuals link themselves to the process at one or more stages.

A role is a pattern of actions expected of a person in recurring situations involving others. Formal roles arise from such factors as one's position in an organization and the technical requirements of work. Informal roles help people to interact with one another in expected ways. Both types of roles provide individuals with a means of anticipating the probable behavior of others and of judging the appropriateness of their own behavior according to the expectations of others.

Role behavior is for the most part relatively inexplicit because individuals perform multiple roles, some of them simultaneously, and because the individual exercises choices not only over which roles to play but how to play them. As individuals gain experience, they learn how to meet the expectations of others in a variety of recurring situations. They come to know what works for them, under what conditions, and when. The development of a role repertory may be largely uncalculated, but it is nevertheless important that administrators be sensitive to the expectations of others, even if they do not respond to them in particular cases.

People in an organization may play a dominant role in certain circumstances, but more commonly they fulfill a number of roles simultaneously or shift as necessary from one role to another.

These roles are not always compatible, although a certain consistency in the performance of roles tends to arise out of habit and of successful experiences that gain the approbation of others. Excessive role conflict can be dysfunctional for the individual as well as for the organization.

Organizationally sensitive individuals cope with bureaucracy by developing a repertory of preferred role behaviors together with the ability to perform an array of roles and to make shifts among them. They know how to get things done in a particular organization and to use the system to get some of the things they want. As one of the vice presidents in Victory Hospital said, "I know how to 'psyche out' the system when I want to put something across."

The cluster of human traits, organizational factors, and professional attitudes comes together in practical settings in the concept of roles. Among these, the change agent role is central. The change agent role is determined in part by internal organizational factors and in part by the mix of inevitable change induced by outside forces impinging on the interlocking nature of the practice of the professions and technologies within the hospital setting.

Most of the managers and employees interviewed at Victory Hospital felt that it was possible to be change agents, but several doubted that it would be desirable or that they could be successful. Highly situational factors, such as the state of the art in a technical field, the habits and beliefs of physicians, the bureaucratic nature of the organization, or pressures from external sources, bear upon the extent of creativity and innovation. To these types of factors must be added the personal attributes of people, such as personality traits, persistence, intelligence, and the motivation to improve.

CHANGE AGENT ROLES IN THE HOSPITAL

Inherent in the role structure of every manager is a certain orientation toward change. There is a cluster of change-related roles known as a role set. These change-related roles relate in turn to more general roles, such as those of supervisor, manager, or administrator.

The predominant role in organization change is that of change agent—one who successfully initiates, executes, or implements change. Related roles are those of innovator, leader, or entrepreneur. Offsetting roles that produce change are those which work against it, such as conserver, resister, or saboteur. These roles do not have a specific, mutually exclusive content; rather, they are terms that indicate a general orientation by which managers may address themselves to problems of change in a variety of ways.

There is no simple, standardized change agent role, since it evolves within its own particular context.

Given appropriate conditions, any individual may be a change agent, but it is important for an organization to provide systematically for the management of change. The hierarchical system of a hospital meets this need through its distribution of authority and responsibility. Thus, the chief administrator is generally expected and empowered to influence change processes through the roles of leader, innovator, or entrepreneur. Vice presidents and professionals do the same but within a narrower range of tasks; department heads and technicians fulfill these needs at operating levels, and hence are even more carefully restricted or constrained. Supervisors and rank-and-file employees are the least influential in initiating and bringing about change.

We will now consider the influence of role behavior innovation and change at four levels of analysis: the chief administrator and the vice presidents, the professionals, the technicians, and the patients.

CHANGE AGENT ROLES AT THE TOP

Mintzberg has classified managerial roles into three categories: interpersonal, informational, and decisional.[1] The change agent role is not cited as such among the ten roles assigned to the three categories. However, three of the roles studied have a bearing on change and innovation: those of leader, monitor, and entrepreneur. In studying the Mintzberg roles in the context of health care organizations, Forrest, Johnson, and Mosher found that, in hospitals, the roles consuming the most time for chief administrators were those of leader, monitor, and entrepreneur. The chief administrators also deemed these three roles as their most important ones. These roles of leader and entrepreneur were also indicated as those they expected to be the most important in the future.[2] From this we may infer that chief administrators generally assign high priority to roles associated with change and innovation. In Victory Hospital, the attitudes of Wright, Ellis, and Watson confirmed this view.

The dominant roles of chief administrators have changed significantly over the years in order to enable them to meet changing internal and external demands. They have changed from business manager (1920s to 1950s), to coordinator (1950s to 1970s), to corporate chief (1970s). An emergent role is that of management team leader—one which is geared to change, growth, and development and to group decisions needed for coping with the increasingly complex demands of the external environment.[3]

In a bureaucracy such as Victory Hospital, the role of innovator is particularly important because there are many circumstances that work against it. The innovator role is lodged principally with the chief administrator. According to Crozier, the role of innovator is the polar figure of the bureaucratic system, and innovation is the most envied achievement, the one for which people are most ready to compete. And since innovation appears primarily at the top and people compete for this role, only a minority of persons can effectively carry it out. Yet people do consciously prepare for the role. Moreover, the innovator role in a bureaucratic system shows special characteristics—the innovator is legislator rather than discoverer. The bureaucratic innovator tries to put everyone in his place and to reorder the world in a better way rather than to launch new patterns or new ways of doing things. [4]

The innovator role at the top is supported by entrepreneurial roles of the second and third echelons of the organization. Persons in these positions can be encouraged to generate and support innovations to achieve rewards, such as promotions, and they will do so if the innovation model at the top encourages them. Indeed, Crozier argues that the freedom and discretion to innovate at the top of a bureaucracy require the action and support of the entrepreneurial groups. The ability to withhold or resist change, while contradictory to their allocated role as change agents in society and in organizations, gives entrepreneurs considerable power over the top echelon administrator. [5]

The higher in the organization, the more explicit becomes the direct assumption of the change agent role. For example, instead of relying on change roles traditionally ascribed to staff units, top line managers forced ideas and change upon them. According to Ellis:

> Staff people here are not idea people; they are the leg
> people. They don't throw out ideas. The personnel
> department for example is clearly our legs. I have
> to think of the idea and then cause them to take the
> actions. They don't identify problems very well.

The influence of a top echelon administrator on change and innovation is further revealed in the attitudes of the Director of Nursing, who felt that it was her responsibility to provide a role model for subordinates. She saw her role as facilitator and teacher as linked to change.

> Winters: I see myself as mainly a facilitator. I'm
> here to help these other people get the work done.

Interviewer: What else is involved in nursing administration?
Winters: Well, I think a lot of it is teaching. The ad-
  ministrator can teach. He should communicate his
  or her experience. For instance, I've been reading
  an interesting book. Have you read Corporation in
  Crisis—Why the Mighty Fall?
Interviewer: No, not yet.
Winters: I have been enjoying it. It tells about how the
  big corporations have become antisocial and how they
  are getting all the power. You ought to read what
  Chrysler has done, for example, or GE or GM.
Interviewer: Do these things apply to your own work?
Winters: Yes, I see a lot of comparisons. I have concluded from this kind of reading that those of us in
  the health care field have got to define our role more
  carefully. We've got to find out what the public wants
  and how to give better service. Whether you are talking about HMOs [health maintenance organizations] or
  expanding community service—we've got to find out
  what's needed and change accordingly. In this kind of
  reading I find that if I substitute the word patient for
  consumer I come out with the same kind of ideas.

The level at which a role is performed has a conditioning effect on the way that role is performed and also upon the performance
of roles at lower levels of the bureaucracy. We have shown, for
example, that Wright, the hospital's chief administrator, was an
aggressive idea man, actively seeking change, but measuring change
proposals against hard economic standards. In early 1975, however, a new administrator, Irving Ross, appeared on the scene.
He viewed his role as that of conserver, consolidating rather than
being a change agent. This portended considerable role adjustment
for managers below him, but it matched the expectations above him
in the Norfield headquarters, which was headed by a conservative
new president who arrived after Ross did. According to Ross:

This is a fascinating place. There are tentacles out
everywhere. There's a lot of complexity here. It's a
unique kind of organization. They're into a lot of things
and there's more here than anybody would suspect.
What's going to be interesting is seeing the organization
get used to a conservative like me. Basically, I'm a
conservative, but people here are used to having a
wheeler-dealer around. I'm pretty sure I'm going to
be different.

During the delay that preceded the filling of the top posts at Victory and at the Norfield headquarters, a number of adjustments were necessary on the part of those remaining in both organizations. In both, but particularly at Victory, management by crisis came to the fore. Long-range planning was crippled. The pace of innovation and change efforts slowed while coping activities increased.

But, in Victory, the coping itself was perceived as having a serendipitous effect on innovation. Nelling, for example, was challenged by the assignment to her of three functional departments formerly under the departed operations vice presidents. She accepted changes in her role because they provided an expansion of her duties:

> Interviewer: What do you think the impact of these continuing vacancies has been on the process of innovation?
> Nelling: Well, I don't think it's been very good for long-range planning. As I say, we have crisis management, putting out fires. So in the sense of being able to develop things to grow and to plan long-run changes, we can't do it. So in that way that kind of innovation is stopped. But in another way the pressure does make us innovative in specific situations. We have to cope with situations and the pressure is likely to push us into some changes in innovation we might not have gone into before.
> Interviewer: How has your job actually changed in the midst of all this other change?
> Nelling: Well, on a temporary basis, the admitting office has been assigned to me, and also the Professional Office Building management and medical records. These are logical assignments because admitting has a direct connection with finance through billing and collecting. Most of our accounts receivable arise from this source, so it is related. Medical records is largely a clerical job and it's logical for me to take over that function. The same is true of the Professional Office Building; it's a matter of finance, primarily. I expect that when the two vice presidential vacancies are finally filled I will still retain these three new functions.

From the comments above, it can be seen that highly innovative activity, such as that possible in long-range planning, shifts to a short-term perspective on innovation because of the need to cope with organization stress. There were general expectations that as soon as a new administrator was appointed, the need for coping strategies would lessen and that organizational stability would be rapidly restored by Ross's appearance on the scene. This process did in fact occur, but not rapidly, since Ross by temperament was more deliberate:

> Interviewer: I am wondering if you are thinking about making any changes here. I know you have two vice presidential vacancies. Are you going to fill them soon?
>
> Ross: I don't know for sure what decisions we'll make. I'm not going to upset everything here and make a lot of fast changes. On the other hand, I'm going to proceed rather carefully to rethink the organizational arrangements. Right now my thinking is that instead of having two vice presidents, with equal status, that I'm going to get one vice president and put all the direct patient activities under him, and an assistant vice president and put a lot of the routine activities under him. That's the way I'm conducting my recruiting at the moment.

As matters turned out, Ross eventually replaced the two operations vice presidents, maintaining the organization essentially the same as it was under Wright.

THE ARTICULATION OF PROFESSIONAL ROLES

One of the common attributes of the professions is the way in which they guard their autonomy, even when associated together in a hospital organization. The resulting insularity of each profession leads to problems of articulation of their roles with respect to one another as well as to patients and employees. Articulation is required where representatives of two or more professionals must work together in a given situation, or when the boundaries separating their respective jurisdictions and responsibilities are not clear-cut. In this study, the roles of physicians, nurses, laboratory technicians, and administrators were found to be interrelated in complex ways and with differing degrees of articulation. Each type of professional was aware of the roles of others, but was able to cope with conflict and to rationalize occasional invasions of areas belonging to others.

One of the most significant professional role interfaces in a hospital is that between staff physicians and the administrators. Typically, such relationships are set up as parallel but separate hierarchies, giving the hospital a bifurcated structure that some consider undesirable organizational practice. Acceptance of the dual structure, however, allows each domain sufficient autonomy to be protected from the other, yet provides a means by which their efforts can be conjoined. Patient care provides a rationalization for each by identifying a common mission. Still, if this system is examined at a deeper level, it becomes apparent that role articulation does not occur without effort, and that gaps and other difficulties may exist. The question of "who really runs this organization" is always present and seldom subject to a clear-cut answer. Moreover, the administrators' view of patients may be different than the physicians' views.

Innovation and change processes shed light on the role performances of physicians and administrators because it is in the management of ideas, innovations, and implementation of change that problems of articulation are most apparent. Roles therefore provide an excellent view of innovation and change.

At Victory, several administrators alluded to difficulties ensuing from the physicians' desire for autonomy and independence. Commenting on his imminent departure from Victory, Wright stated that:

> It's going to be quite a change in some ways but very similar in other ways. You see, a lot of it has to do with my philosophy and outlook on things. As a hospital administrator, I find that one of our biggest problems is the strong feeling on the part of physicians and surgeons that they have to be independent. They highly value their independence and a one-to-one relationship with patients and other people. They don't really work as a team. It's hard for the patient who has a complaint to know where to go first. We don't have enough general practitioners, family physicians, and that sort of thing. What we need is a better referral system by family or general practitioner physicians. I believe in people and I think we should think about people first and let the organization take second place. Here there is no good way for me to bring that about.

The desire of physicians for independence is in effect achieved as an overt role posture. All the vice presidents indicated that "physicians are not really part of our organization." Yet some physicians were at least loosely attached to the organization structure, though their actual relationships were ambiguous. Asked whether any physicians reported directly to administrators, Wright indicated that "it was a case of both yes and no":

There are some MDs in administrative positions in
the hospital but it is purely convenience and a technical matter, since medical expertise controls most of
the critical decisions and for all practical purposes
they are set apart from the regular administrative
staff.

In this study it was not possible to interview Victory's physicians generally, but three physician department heads were interviewed—radiology, pathology, and anesthesiology. The physician-
administrator has been too little studied by both health care and
management researchers. Here it is possible to suggest only some
tentative conclusions about role sets of physician-administrators
with respect to their influence on innovation and change.

In the dual roles of "physician" and "administrator," that of
physician remains dominant. Physician autonomy is preserved by
(1) careful role differentiation and (2) keeping administrative duties
at a minimum level. They stressed their work with and relationships to their patients. They also set up their own private corporations, in effect contracting their services to Victory. They also
delegated administrative responsibilities heavily to chief technicians
or clerical personnel. For example, the chief of staff at the time
of this research was also the head of one of the laboratories. This
led to heavy reliance on a medical secretary for chief of staff
functions.

The anesthesiologists and the physicians in pathology and in
radiology were organized as corporations. The hospital furnished
space, supplies, and equipment. Patients were billed separately for
hospital costs and physicians' fees. The head of the pathology group
received a salary based on a percentage of the income generated by
the laboratory. In general, the corporations hire their own clinical
and technical employees. This causes patient confusion over billings. One physician described this problem as follows:

The patient gets two bills, one for the use of the hospital and one from the doctor for his fee. A lot of
times patients don't understand this and they are
shocked to get two different bills. As long as we have
a fee-for-service system, this will happen, but no
matter how carefully we explain things they are still
surprised.

The physician-administrators expressed no clear view of their
possible roles as innovators or change agents. Instead, they viewed
cooperation with other administrators as highly important, for

ultimately it was the general administrators who approved or re-jected the changes they desired. The physician-administrators had strong views of the changes they wanted. They provided information to support their case, but otherwise did not actively pursue change through the usual change agent processes of give-and-take in the political-administrative process. Some desired changes were assumed to win eventual approval because of their merit and the professional endorsement of physicians. Other desired changes, such as "the need for more space in our lab," were not actively pursued because there appeared to be little hope of attaining them.

Thus, cooperation with the hospital's administrators was the strategy underlying the physician-administrators' pursuit of change. They regarded this relationship with hospital personnel as generally amicable, mutually beneficial, and satisfactory. According to the head of anesthesiology:

> There are a lot of ways in which we work together. We cooperate a lot on teaching. For example, the hospital finances the stipends for nurse anesthetist students in their first year, and we pay their stipends at later stages of their training. Another example of the cooperation is that the nurse anesthetist is on call 24 hours a day, mainly for obstetrical cases. We pay the nurses a salary, but when there is something like a Code Blue alert, a cardiac arrest, they can call on our nurse anesthetists for help. They also help out in the emergency room. The hospital pays our firm for each delivery that our nurses are called in on. So both the hospital and our firm get in on things like this.

Nurses at Victory, however, saw the need for greater collabo-ration between administrators and physicians as an important prob-lem. They felt that nurses can be an instrument of improved rela-tionships between them through a catalyst role. According to the vice president of nursing:

> We need a great deal more cohesiveness between doc-tors and administrators. I think the nurse is a catalyst between doctors and administrators. I don't think you are ever going to have administrators bringing the doctors to them or the doctors bringing the administra-tors to them. I think the nurse is in the most strategic spot to bring them together.

Physicians at Victory were very much aware of social pres-sures in their profession. These social pressures have an impact on the physician-administrator relationships because the physician, not the patient, is the true client of the hospital. Social pressures, such as requirements for PSRO (Professional Standards Review Organizations) audits, the greater use of paramedicals, pressures on costs, and demands for increased services and better equipment, ultimately extend to the administrators of the hospital and to the staffs those administrators supervise.

As social pressures portend change, they have potentials for increasing the conflict and stress between the physician and administrator roles. One of the physician-administrators, for example, believed that the need for mediating social pressures would increase the influence of the administrators over that of physicians:

> Physician: Well, one change I can tell you about . . . is that whether they know it or not and whether they like it or not, the administrators are making policy for the medical side of things. I know they are not supposed to, and nobody likes it, but there's no use kidding, that's what's actually going on. I think part of it is coming from the government. We have these PSRO audits now, for example, and that's only a part of it.
>
> Interviewer: Would the administrators admit that they are doing this or do you think they would deny it?
>
> Physician: They would probably deny it because they are not supposed to be doing it. It's not their fault. They don't do it too directly. Of course they can't interfere in any actual medical decision but they come around and say, "Have you thought about so and so?" "If you don't do such and such, it's going to interfere with the collection of our third-party payments and you know we will all suffer if that happens." So there are pressures on the administrators coming from a lot of complex parts of the system and it is causing them to interfere more in the policy side of medical work than before.
>
> Interviewer: I see.
>
> Physician: Another reason we have some conflict between physicians and the administrators is that we don't have any positions on the board of trustees. It's true, no administrator votes on the board either, but they are closer all the time and work with them much more than we get to. We need to have a voice on the board. We hate to beg, there's no use in getting up hollering and raving and ranting all the time, but we have

hollered to become voting members and I think it's a good thing we did, although nothing has been done yet.

The same physician also reported a problem of differential respect, again emphasizing the added social pressure of governmental interference:

> Interviewer: Why do you think conflict has increased between physicians and administrators?
> Physician: I'm not sure I know the answer but I suspect partly because we are here in the South. Up North, they have had traditions of respect for each other. In the South, we're the last to get respect. Also, I think there's the interference of the government in everything we do and that is bringing us into conflict.

Another physician saw social pressures as attacking the principle of physicians' autonomy and independence through a breakdown in the fee-for-service system:

> There are a few changes in radiology coming up, as I think they are getting some new equipment. There is a big rhubarb in pathology. It's going on here right now. Their doctors are on salary and they want to be independent. They are fighting with the administration right now and there is going to be a crunch on that. Also, it may be that we'll have some organizational changes. It may not be possible to be independent contractors any more with a fee for service. There is too much social pressure, though a lot of it is misinformed. . . . When you think about patient rights and other patient demands, I think people have promised too much. That's one thing that is driving costs up. They don't have any regard for cost but we have to keep trying to meet patient demand.

RESISTANCE TO CHANGE

Embodied in the role conflicts we have described is the factor of resistance to change. While role conflict does not explain all the factors related to resistance, it seems particularly appropriate in examining interprofessional relationships in the hospital. Roles among professionals reveal a strong element of domain consciousness arising from considerations of autonomy, authority, and status.

The relations among anesthesiologists, physicians' assistants, and nurse anesthetists are illustrative. Some anesthesiologists at Victory were largely opposed to physicians' assistants. But the anesthesiologists throughout the country have also considered eliminating nurse anesthetists. There is a paradox here, in that they oppose even physicians' assistants who would presumably be under closer physician control than would members of the more independent and better established nursing profession. One of the anesthesiologists at Victory described the situation as follows:

> There are only two or three schools in the whole country training physicians' assistants in anesthetics, but these programs have been called to a halt. So many anesthesiologists were against it, as I am. First the American Society of Anesthesiologists had hoped to supplant all nurses with physicians. You can see this was an unrealistic dream, that we could never train enough to do it. Here we have the reverse of the British system. In Britain only a physician can give an anesthetic, but they use midwives for delivering babies. In the United States, we have both physicians and nurses giving anesthetics, but only an M. D. can be an obstetrician so we decided in the society that we can't bury the nurses. We've decided to cooperate with them and get along with them. So we have ways of getting together frequently with them. For example, nurse anesthetists are invited to our meetings.

In these views we see the possibility that in resisting the advent of physicians' assistants, physicians are in effect resisting role proliferation. That is, they have long-established role relationships with nurse anesthetists. They see little need for complicating their work with still another group competing for a standing in the hierarchy. Both groups are examples of an innovation that received great impetus and approval in early stages, but which eventually faded because there appeared to be no effective way of ameliorating potential role conflicts. Social pressures were evidently not sufficient to support these innovations. According to one of the anesthesiologists:

> Anesthesiology is pretty much shielded from the pressures, but . . . the anesthetist is not in the foreground of patient awareness. Also, he is not among the top ten in the status rankings of the prestige poll in the paramedic association . . . but he isn't at the bottom either.

Also, in malpractice suits, the anesthesiologist was in
the number one group with the neurosurgeons and ortho-
pedic surgeons. Fortunately, the anesthesiologists has
now dropped down to the number two position along with
plastic surgeons and obstetricians. But I do think that
the criticism is leveled against medicine as a whole,
rather than against us as anesthesiologists.

Professionals, even more so than technicians, have difficulty
in articulating their professional roles with their administrative
and change agent roles. It was surprising to find that some key
managers at Victory were uncomfortable in their administrative
roles, yet comfortable in their change agent roles. This was due
in part to their distaste for managerial roles, since this represents
an abandonment of original career choices, the decline of their
technical expertness, involvement in matters where their skills
are less developed, and the need to deal with trivia that nonmanager
professionals can reject. It was also due to the fact that they viewed
change more as "the ability to work with people" than as a managerial process. An example is Winters, who expressed strong
rejection of the administrative role and a high level of concern for
the clinical role. Yet she was a dynamic performer of her change
agent role:

> Winters: I just love change. I want things to move.
> I'd rather be a director of nursing like I was and be
> able to make some things happen. As it is I'm all
> tied up in the bureaucracy. . . . Changing to vice
> president did not involve too much real change in my
> job role, but I don't like the changes that did happen.
> Interviewer: What were these changes like?
> Winters: Well, I attend a lot of meetings I didn't have to
> go to before. Most of my time is involved with the
> people higher up. I meet once a week with all the
> vice presidents of administration. I meet with a joint
> council of physicians and trustees quarterly, that's
> for the whole Norfield Medical Complex. I don't go
> to the executive meetings of physicians but the other
> vice presidents do. I don't really care. I don't want
> to go to their meetings. I accomplished a lot more
> when I was Director of Nursing than before I got so
> involved with bureaucracy.

THE ROLES OF TECHNICIANS

A whole new set of role relationships is evolving in the modern hospital. These were most evident in Victory Hospital, where technicians were observed to be developing roles that more closely link them with physicians, nurses, and administrators. These new roles tend to elevate the status, prestige, and importance of technicians; they point the technician toward a greater professionalism; they make possible for the technician a larger role in innovation and change. The new roles also increase the potential for role conflict, since the extension of the technician's role collides with the roles of the traditional professions. Technicians display aspirations which cannot help but intervene in the established protocols and pecking orders.

As technicians interact with physicians, nurses, and administrators, they are gradually able to assume some of the role behaviors formerly ascribed to these other groups. Thus, in addition to their technical roles, they may acquire therapeutic roles from nurses or physicians, and if appointed to an administrative position, they acquire additional roles in this sector. To the extent that these roles are not congruent, the technician experiences conflict, tension, and stress in meeting the expectations of others. Members of the related groups, too, may experience tensions resulting from changes in their roles.

Change at Victory has involved to a considerable degree the acquisition by technicians of roles and duties formerly ascribed to higher-level professionals, such as nurses. The development of the cardiovascular laboratory, for example, involved the transfer of certain patient care procedures from nurses to technicians. This devolution of responsibility, however, resulted in an increased status for cardiovascular technicians. Not only was their responsibility increased by this change but they were also brought into closer patterns of interaction with physicians and their potential for role conflict was intensified. According to the head of the cardiovascular laboratory:

> Some people might consider it rather strange that we don't have x-ray technicians in the catheterization lab. We do our own x-rays. When I first came to Victory, the catheterization lab didn't exist as it does today. It was run by nurses and they were doing six or eight a month. The nurses weren't technically oriented and I think this is what I brought into the picture. . . .
> The reason we have such an efficient cardiovascular technician unit here is that we assume so much

responsibility. For example, in a typical operating
room in most hospitals you find certain people doing
only certain jobs and none really sensitive or really
responsible for maintenance. However, in our OR you
don't see nurses standing around administering drugs.
The cardiovascular technician has taken this responsibility. Now it means more work for us, but it also
motivates our people to put more of themselves into it
because we know the patient is relying on us. Also,
legally we may be out on a limb in some of the responsibility we have taken on as technicians. I think this
helps to motivate the people in the unit here to do a
good job because if anything ever did go wrong there
could be problems.

The head of the cardiovascular laboratory also indicated the
multiple roles of the technicians and the importance of the relative
knowledge and skills apportioned among physicians, surgeons,
nurses, and technicians:

Our people are actually trained to be part doctor's
assistant, part surgeon's assistant, and part technician. We know more about pharmacology, the administering of medicine, and physiology than most
nurses and I think the doctors here will agree with
that. Our job is to take care of the patient, and here
in the cardiovascular lab we welcome the responsibility. In our atraumatic or noninvasive lab we do echo
studies of the patients. . . . We're left more or less
on our own. However, the doctors really oversee our
work. . . . This I imagine has its good and bad sides,
the good side being that the doctor doesn't have to
worry about it and leaves him free to do other things
more important. On the other hand, the bad side is
the potential for error which I think we have effectively
minimized.

The following comments of the head of the cardiovascular laboratory indicate that the interface between technicians and physicians
is a difficult one:

Back in 1968 before I started working here I was still
in school learning to be a pump technician and realized
the potential that echo studies might have for the type
of work that I was doing. Therefore, I learned on my

own, self-taught so to speak, and really at that time
nobody knew anything about echo studies. Now, there
are a lot of physicians who know a lot more than I do.
However, I still know quite a bit and I'm still left on
my own to do this type of work. As a matter of fact,
there have been times when I have felt a little uncomfortable that I was talking about such a technical area
with doctors. This is traditionally an area that doctors
specialize in and no one else knows much about. Anyhow, I felt uncomfortable because I wasn't a doctor.
But I can converse with practically anybody on the
subject.

As a result of the interplay of role behaviors among physicians,
nurses, and technicians and their link to administrative roles, the
question of role congruence arises. Role congruence is the extent
to which the expectations within multiple roles can be met with a
minimum of dissonance or conflict. If technical, professional, and
administrative roles are incongruent, it becomes difficult to play
the additional role of change agent. Ultimately, the change agent
cannot act alone. He must persuade others to want what he wants.
He has to acquire a position of trust, power, status, and respect
among peers, subordinates, and superiors.

Technicians at Victory benefited from a special mechanism
designed to enhance their standing as "professionals." This system
confers professional status on a department in the hospital. This
status had to be earned, but the basis for earning it was peculiar:
being able to generate a certain level of income. This in turn
caused departments seeking this status to demand extensive records
and documentation to support their case for professional standing
in the hospital. According to the data control coordinator:

To achieve professional status for a department means
to be recognized by the hospital or the administration
as being professional as opposed to being technical or
semiprofessional. The main result . . . is the benefit
that can accrue to the individual department or group,
such as pay raises. Now I'm not exactly sure what all
the prerequisites are for being recognized on a professional status, but I do know one is the fact that the unit
has to be able to show that it is generating X amount of
dollars. The best way to do this is to keep accurate
and extensive revenue and cost reports. That's where
I enter into the picture. Some groups such as radiology,
clinical laboratories, and the cardiovascular group have

what is called professional components. That is, the
whole group has not achieved this professional status
but is recognized because they perform certain jobs and
generate, as I mentioned, X amount of dollars. By the
way, groups that achieve this classification can also
charge additional fees. Recently our inhalation therapy
department has been trying to get this recognition and
therefore they've been collecting a lot of information
from my department. I understand that inhalation
therapy has been recognized in other hospitals in this
city for this professional status.

In many instances at Victory, there was substantial perceived
incongruence between the technicians' roles as technicians compared to their roles as administrators (department heads). When a
technician becomes the manager of a group of other technicians,
others hold expectations that he will perform managerial tasks while
at the same time continuing to meet their technical expectations.

The hospital, like other organizations, has a two-track system for the advancement of one's career: a promotion ladder in
management responsibility and one in the functional or technical
fields. At some point the individual selects a preferred route of
advancement. Many technical or professional people who follow
the managerial career ladder can adjust to the parallel roles only
with considerable effort. They ultimately experience difficulty and
disappointment from the inevitable decline of their technical or
professional skills, although this depends heavily on their earlier
commitments to their field of interest, as well as on their degree
of success in them. In any case, the roles may become increasingly
incongruent until a firm commitment one way or the other can develop. This type of role incongruence can be illustrated by a comment of the chief radiological technician:

When I first came here I was still trying to hold on to
my technical work. I was doing eight hours a day of
cobalt therapy. Then suddenly Mr. Wright caught on
to what I was doing. I was enjoying patient contact.
That's what I got into this work in the first place for,
but Mr. Wright was very firm about this. He said as
soon as therapy got to be more than 50 percent of my
time that I had to get a therapy technician. So after a
year I gave up all technical work. I finally got my first
technician and was down to 50 percent and then in a year
gave it all up. I can see now Mr. Wright was correct,
but I hated to give it up. Four years after I became

full-time administrator, I got a chief assistant. She
helps manage the other technicians and helps around
the office. Some people bypass the assistant and come
directly to me. I didn't want to keep them from doing
that. There's no ciriticism if people come directly to
me, but the assistant can run a lot of our activities for
me and that helps me make better use of my time.

The chief technician's adjustment to the change from technical
skills was further explained as follows:

A lot of people here fell by the wayside when we moved
from the old location. They were the ones who couldn't
learn to adjust or to change. They wanted to go on
doing things the same old way and they are no longer
here. I admit that I have a lot of limitations. I'm not
a college graduate, for example. I only have a two-
year technician's degree. Also, I've lost my technical
ability. I don't know a lot about techniques and some
of them I couldn't even demonstrate for you anymore.
In fact I was so concerned about this I went to Mr. Wright
and told him that I couldn't help the technicians anymore
technically. He said he didn't care, that that was no
longer part of my job. However, it worried me. I
thought I had better tell him about it rather than have
him bring somebody through here sometime and have
him learn that way that I couldn't explain what was
going on. I couldn't stand wondering how he felt so
I had to discuss this with him.

Similarly, the head of the cardiovascular laboratory indicated
considerable tension between his administrative and technical roles
and the importance of his teaching role:

To be honest, I don't consider myself to be much of an
administrator. Really, my philosophy is that I am a
technician first. I feel that this is really a functional
attitude to the uniqueness of our department because we
cover so many areas. We have to cross-train everybody, and since I know more than anyone in my department I am responsible personally for the teaching function per se. . . . I'm sort of alien to department head
meetings; as a matter of fact I haven't been to one in
over a year, since we got two cardiologists. However,
I feel my primary job is patient maintenance. Therefore,

if I'm too busy to take care of my administrative detail,
luckily my boss understands that I'm a technician first
and there's not any conflict.

The roles of medical technicians vis-à-vis the roles of administrators and physicians are also complex. The technicians
appeared to view their role as primarily a professional responsibility for the care of patients and the performance of technical duties
no one else, such as the physicians, knows how to perform. They
expressed a reluctance to accept administrative duties, such as
running a laboratory. They also indicated an appreciation of problems of intercommunication between themselves and the physicians
and administrators. For example, the head of the department of
physical therapy reported that:

> . . . I'm kept very busy because not only am I the
> supervisor . . . I also have to administer physical
> therapy to patients. Therefore, I don't have as much
> time to be a supervisor and administer to the depart-
> ment as I'd like to. One of my responsibilities is
> scheduling the work of our physical therapists. . . .
> Another of my responsibilities is interpreting doctors'
> orders and checking out the exact procedure to admin-
> ister. . . . Another of my primary responsibilities in
> the hospital is the teaching function. Also I conduct
> orientations for groups as they pass through the depart-
> ment. These groups include administration and minis-
> terial. They usually expect nothing more than a little
> talk on our objectives and purposes and goals. Another
> of my supervisory responsibilities . . . is to commu-
> nicate with doctors. For example, last year we did a
> booklet on the available modality and treatment deemed
> useful in specific types of disorders. This was done
> primarily for the doctors' information because some
> doctors don't really become exposed to physical therapy
> in their academic training.

Technicians are often caught up in conflicts in the form of resistance to change by professionals such as nurses or physicians.
For example, an operations vice president instructed the head of
the maintenance department to make certain modifications of physical arrangements in the operating rooms. The physician thus
affected resisted the changes, putting the head of maintenance on
the spot. He wrote a memo to Ellis and asked for a discussion with
him, rather than pursuing his case directly with the physicians.

On some issues he indicated a willingness to talk with physicians, but only if it would not result in any embarrassment to Ellis, whom he believed should be kept fully informed. In clarifying his views, he indicated considerable disdain for confrontations with physicians, explaining that he was protected from them by the chain of command:

> Really, I don't have to give the doctor the time of day. They are not in my chain of command and I'm not responsible to them and they are not responsible for decisions I make. The board and the administration are responsible for situations like this. The medical staff members of this hospital have inputs into the administrative system at a higher level than I'm on. Like I said, I can interact with them but I don't have to.

Another example of role conflict was found between the work of the dietary department and nurses. All feeding of patients, employees, and visitors was under the control of the dietary department. But 3 percent of the patients have special requirements, so that nurses must carry their trays. Nurses resented this work and the dietary staff felt that the nurses did not perform these functions well. According to the head of the dietary department, they lost trays, patients weren't served, and food was wasted.

The difficulties between the dietary department and nursing continued despite liaison meetins designed to improve communication. According to its head:

> Usually nursing and dietary get along fairly well. We have a liaison meeting once a month in which three dieticians meet with three nurses on the committee and the problems are aired. I feel that since basically our objectives are the same, that is, serving the patients, there is incentive for nursing and dietary to work together in a coordinated manner. However, this system is not perfect. For instance, a lot of times our communications will get crossed up because a nurse forgot to put a dietary change on the chart or maybe forgot to tell us that a patient was not supposed to have a meal. Consequently, we've learned to listen to the patient. If the patient says, for instance, that she is not supposed to have a meal, we won't argue with the patient. We'll go to the nursing staff and find out if it is true. Most of the time the patient knows what he's talking about.

PATIENT ROLES AND THE INNOVATION PROCESS

The widespread overt acceptance of many hospital employees of high quality patient care as their central raison d'être raises interesting questions for an examination of innovation and change. For example, are the frequent allusions to the patient care objective merely lip service to an idealized, public image concept? Do patient care objectives play a significant part in generating innovation and change? If patient care is an energizing, motivating force in the work of hospital personnel, it should be an instrumental force in innovation and change.

At Victory Hospital, patient care appeared to be an anchoring concept, a central reference point for the collaborative efforts of the members of the organization. It provided a common, often overriding, frame of reference. Such a fact, however, should not be permitted to mask the complexities inherent in the conduct of organization members carrying out their daily responsibilities. A given patient, for example, receives care from many persons, both seen and unseen. But it is the nature of the direct contacts which are most likely to influence the patient's attitudes and evaluations of the care received. The patient can ultimately judge the results of his hospital stay by how he feels and whether or not he is "cured" or on the way toward improvement. Moreover, the degree of direct personal interaction between a patient and the hospital's staff members varies by function, by level of organization, by patient needs, by the professional competencies and attitudes of the staff members, and by the personality configurations of patients. For those whose contacts with patients are relatively indirect, patient care dicta are less persuasive. Yet everything may count in the final result.

Additional complications arise from the patient's difficulty in distinguishing clearly between the room service, hotel functions and those more directly related to health or medical services. Patients expect to be hurt or inconvenienced by diagnostic and therapeutic procedures, but these are more tolerable when accompanied by effectively managed hospital facilities. Thus, patients may accept the ministrations of physicians, nurses, and technicians on faith, but have strong opinions on how the hospital's staff and facilities affect them.

Just as patient care provides an anchoring concept for many if not most hospital employees, the physician's role also anchors their behavior, since patient care is at the center for the physician as well. The physician thus provides a role model that can demonstrate to other professionsals, semiprofessionals, and technicians

the meaning of patient care. These twin anchors—patient care and
the physician as a role model—give direction and guidance to the
processes of innovation and change, but they also provide limits:
a change not in the patient's interest, or without benefit to the patient, or a change not approved by physicians, will tend not to occur.

This leads to the problem of determining what the effects of a
proposed change may be on the physicians and on patients. Where
costs are not determining, so that a "purely administrative" decision can be made, judgment must be used. In this realm, opinions
of knowledgeable persons often differ. The uncertainties in predicting the effects of change will reinforce the tendency to maintain
the status quo. Furthermore, in the absence of concrete concepts
of quality for patient care, both those favoring and those opposing
change may resort to patient care arguments.

In the hospital, patients submit themselves to hospital routines
and the ministrations of nurses, physicians, and technicians. Service requirements are highly personal and individualized for each
patient. The patient's role consists of two facets: accommodation
to hospital norms for "the good patient," and the receiver and
evaluator of the quality of care provided.

Both role facets are subservient in character. The good
patient follows instructions, does what he is told, and raises a
minimum of questions and complaints. As a receiver and evaluator of care, he has no explicit medical or other professional criteria to apply. He only knows how he feels, whether he is better
or worse, and some general attitudes about quality of care.

The patient does not realize that even professionals cannot
identify explicit measures of the quality of care. Nevertheless, in
Victory Hospital, staff members having close contact with patients
were found to have a strong feeling about their missions with respect to the problem of quality care for patients. For example,
according to a unit coordinator in nursing:

> As you are probably aware, there is no true measure
> of quality care, none that everyone feels is really
> accurate today. We spent two years writing a "stan-
> dards of care" manual. We had a consulting firm study
> quality control. The results of the study were that
> several standards were identified among this hospital
> and about 13 others across the United States and these
> norms or averages were used to rate our hospital. We
> came out real high on leadership. The results of the
> study are not what really gave me these ideas. As a
> matter of fact, the results were vague to me and until
> this day I don't understand them. However, the methods

and processes they used to compile their data were interesting and I have been using them personally. . . .
I started asking patients more questions personally
when I made my rounds. I became more sensitive as
to how our care was coming across to the patient. I
know that patients are sometimes reluctant to criticize
the nursing staff and when they are critical they often
ask me to not tell their particular nurse because they
don't want any reprisals. Of course, this is just ig-
norance on their part, but the point is there were some
valid criticisms. I decided, therefore, to try to quantify
some of these patient feelings, and asked my nursing
staff to come up with a few questions. This resulted in
38 questions. I plan on picking out maybe ten of the best
and compiling them into a survey for the patient to fill
out. Then we can get some feedback from patients on
what kind of care we are giving. We once tried sending
out letters to patients and even put a stamp on the return
envelope. However, the patients . . . just didn't mail
the letters back.

Within the limits of this study, it was not possible to make a
detailed study of patients or staff physicians. However, nine patient interviews were obtained, only two of which with former
patients at Victory. A semistructured interview schedule was constructed by which the person interviewed was asked for opinions
comparing the latest hospital stay to the previous stays. The
questions were open-ended, inviting patients to comment freely.

The patients were interviewed from a few weeks to not more
than two years after their hospital stay. Only some general observations are possible, but they do shed light on patient awareness
of innovation and change. In sum, these interviews tend to indicate
that hospitalization has improved as medical treatment has improved,
and so have administrative processes such as admitting, billing,
and other office procedures. Patients reported an improvement in
"the professional handling of the hospital stay." That is, procedures
in the office are more efficient today than in the past.

It is more difficult for the patient to evaluate changes in medical practice. For example, one patient recalled differences in
procedures for heart patients in 1968 as compared to 1974. His first
heart attack in 1968 resulted in a hospital stay of 22 days and a total
of 90 days' loss of work. In 1974, the same patient had heart surgery which resulted in missing only six weeks of work. Also, he
was ambulated less than 48 hours after his operation. While early
ambulation and other self-help procedures devolving on patients are

no doubt medically sound, patients are likely to judge these as deficiencies in the hospital's overall care.

Several patients saw hospitalization as being more impersonal and that one has to "do for yourself" much more now. Two of these interviewed could see no change in recent hospitalizations. One remarked that "hospitalization today is the same as it was 10 to 15 years ago." Although changes and new developments are constantly being made in hospitals today, patients may not be aware that changes are occurring. One patient who was an administrator for the hospital in which he stayed, could not remember any new developments or procedures that occurred while he was a patient. However, he held administrative meetings in his room and noted that there was an informality directed toward him. Another patient observed that serving food had gotten "too mechanical." Another discovered that the hospital had what they called a VIP list. This person felt that being on this list caused the nurses to resent him: "It was as if they went out of their way to make life hard." However, unless changes directly affect the patient, he is generally unaware of them.

A majority of the patients interviewed found the admitting process to be very good. One patient estimated that the process took only 45 minutes. This the patient considered a "record time." The longest wait for admission was nearly three hours. Those who gave a "poor" rating to the admitting process did so partly because of long waits in the lobby, or because of errors on the forms. One patient thought that in addition to procedures being unorganized, the "drill sergeant technique" of the person who handled the admitting was a problem. While patients did not consciously note that the admitting process was more efficient today because of new developments such as computers, they did experience improvements, as shown by the favorable ratings they gave.

Patients found no great differences in their most recent hospital stay as compared to former stays in hospitals. The general consensus was that things were about equal. Only one patient described his most recent stay as "the worst I've had." This particular patient based this opinion largely on the treatment and services received from the nursing staff. For example, one of the LPNs on duty was a "pure deadbeat," sitting around reading the paper when she should have administered medication. Instead, she waited until the RN came back to do it. Three specific things that accounted for this "very poor" rating were: "total indifference, incompetence on the part of the nursing staff, and the filthiness of the place." By contrast, another patient saw his stay as better than any former stays in terms of providing good service, information, and good admitting and discharging processes.

Because the majority of patients could not recall any great differences in their most recent stay and former hospital stays, it is possible that they tend either to categorize their hospital stays as ordinary and routine, or they tend to block out any perceived differences. Those with strongly negative attitudes toward their stays could usually point to specific unsatisfactory events.

Five of the patients interviewed said that they did not receive all the information they wanted in a timely manner. In some instances, patients received the wrong information. For example, in one case, a patient asked how long he would be placed on a respirator. He was told that it would "be for a few hours, maybe four." As it turned out, he was placed on the machine for 21 hours.

Patients seem to resent most of all the fact that they were not kept informed about what was going on or why something was being done. A hospital's policy of withholding information from a patient may be grounded in a desire to keep the patient from becoming alarmed or frightened. However, the patient tends to feel that he can handle a certain amount of information, and not knowing only adds to his fears. As one patient put it, "There is a fine line between educating and causing great consternation or fear."

Only two out of the nine people interviewed were familiar with the "Patient's Bill of Rights." In none of the hospitals concerned, including Victory, was the Bill of Rights actually in effect. The Patient's Bill of Rights, treating such matters as the information given to the patient, discriminatory acts, explanations of billing, care and treatment procedures, refusal of services, and the like has been promulgated by the American Hospital Association to over 7,000 hospitals in the United States. A number of government agencies have contemplated issuing similar dicta. But it remains an innovation that is slow to take hold.

Another innovation that has not become widespread was instituted by an Ohio hospital—a guarantee of patient satisfaction, "or your money back." In the first year, $12,000 was budgeted for refunds, but less than $150 had to be returned. [6]

Surgery in a hospital without a hospital stay has increased markedly in the United States. This innovation involves setting up a special unit for quick processing of patients requiring only minor surgery. A survey by the American Hospital Association in 1973 showed that 1,427 of the nation's 7,000 hospitals had such units. No specific effort in this direction was found in Victory Hospital, although its administrators were exploring all aspects of outpatient care during the time of this study. A nearby investor-owned hospital advertises "same-day surgery."

IDEALISM AND HEALTH CARE ROLES

The inherent nature of a bureaucracy precludes undefined, open-ended roles. Yet even within a highly structured bureaucracy such as Victory Hospital, individuals may have a wide latitude in the way they perform their roles. Yet for many the ideal is never attained. The expectations to which roles respond are often beyond the individual's capabilities of meeting them. It is one of the functions of professionalism to hold before the individual an ideal image of what behavior the roles should take. This striving for the ideal mandates a posture for innovation and change.

The interacting roles of physicians, administrators, professionals, technicians, and patients merit more research than they have as yet received. In this chapter, we have illustrated various aspects of these roles as they bear upon innovation and change. More attention should be paid to the management processes whereby hospital employees and medical staffs address themselves to the human aspects of the patient care process. Those patients who have severely criticized hospital care have done so largely because of deficiencies in the human relations orientation of hospital and professional personnel, not because of the technical procedures, apparatus, and capabilities of medical services.[7]

Technical or medical innovation has made substantial progress as it is carried out in hospitals. It is management's task to link these forms of progress to patient needs by innovation and change in the managerial sphere. It is in this latter responsibility that today's hospitals are woefully deficient.

NOTES

1. Henry Mintzberg, "A New Look at the Chief Executive's Job," Organizational Dynamics, Winter 1973, pp. 20-30; "The Manager's Job: Folklore and Fact," Harvard Business Review 53 (July-August 1975): 49-61.
2. Christopher R. Forrest, Alton C. Johnson, and John Mosher, "A Profile of the Health Organization Chief Executive Officer," in Academy of Management, 37th Annual Proceedings, ed. Robert L. Taylor et al., 1977.
3. See Rockwell Shultz and Alton C. Johnson, Management of Hospitals (New York: McGraw-Hill, 1976), Ch. 9.
4. Michel Crozier, The Bureaucratic Phenomenon (Chicago: University of Chicago Press, 1964), p. 201.
5. Ibid., p. 202.

6. Newsweek, December 29, 1975, p. 52.

7. See, for example, Irvine H. Page, M.D., "Why Patients Love Their Patience," Modern Medicine, April 1, 1975, p. 9; and Charles D. Aring, M.D., "Obsolescence in the Hospital," Journal of the American Medical Association, June 10, 1974, pp. 1393-94.

11

RESISTANCE: THE LIMITS OF
INNOVATION AND CHANGE

The feedback model of innovation and change we have been exploring in this book describes a process which can be interrupted at any point. One type of interruption is based on logical analysis, testing, and evaluation leading to rational decisions to abort or discontinue proposed changes. This way of preventing change was explored in Chapter 8.

Another way in which change and innovation may be halted or prevented consists of more subtle resistance strategies which infiltrate the logical processes of change. Those who oppose change or revere the status quo may combat it by logical or rational means where possible, but the real significance of resistance to change lies in the emotional and attitudinal factors which underlie the behavior of people at work.

Change in hospitals is a difficult process. Not only is there resistance by people, but the system of health care of which hospitals are a fundamental part can also be restrictive to change. Some problems in a hospital persist because elements in the larger system are slow to change. And within a hospital such as Victory, the complexity of the organization and its problems serves to make any significant change slow and difficult.

A successful change is the product of many forces at work inside and outside the hospital; it is the resultant of a balance tipped in one direction or another by a variety of strategies and circumstances. In Victory, as in most organizations, a successful change has to overcome enormous odds. As Herbert Kaufman has observed, a substantial change is an improbable occurrence, since bureaucratization tends to reinforce stability.[1] In Victory, Vice President Ellis believed that factors tending against innovation and change outweigh the favorable tendencies:

> I think there are many factors affecting the process,
> but on balance there are more deterrents than motivat-
> ing factors. For example, one of my pet peeves is
> third-party funding. Third-party funding deters our
> outpatient service expansion. We have a fine facility
> here, and a good organization, but why can't we be
> more aggressive and energetic in the whole health
> care field? It's dollars entirely. We get pretty good
> coverage for inpatient care, but it's ridiculous for
> the outpatient services.

Ellis's perceptions contrast starkly with the aggressive, expansionist tendencies within Victory and its parent organization,
Norfield. Beds were increased in number even though there was a
900-bed surplus in the community as a whole. Expensive equipment, such as a scanner, was added despite its duplication in three
other hospitals nearby. Clearly technical changes that can be justified on a cost-revenue basis can be achieved against great odds by
persistent administrative drive if supported by physicians and if
strategies are available for overcoming limitations imposed by public agencies.

Administrative change comes with greater difficulty. The
administrative drive that puts over a technological or physical
change does not work as well for administrative change. Instead,
leadership and persuasion are needed, for power plays or sheer
coercion engender resistance and alienate those slated to carry out
the change. These difficulties explain in part at least the continuous
feeling of dissatisfaction about the pace of change expressed by Ellis:

> It's hard to change anything in a hospital. For one
> thing, you have too many outsiders involved. You
> have a lot of groups watching what you're doing and
> getting concerned over the effects of change on them.
> Almost always we have to hold a decision up for sev-
> eral weeks after it's been made just to collect in
> those reactions and to see what else we ought to
> change in the plan. Everybody wants a say and this
> makes for a delay. You've got 500 doctors around
> here, for example, and they're not even on the pay-
> roll but they have a lot of say. Or we might get com-
> plaints from nursing and so allow some delays while
> we seek ideas.

PATTERNS OF RESISTANCE TO CHANGE

Patterns of resistance may be seen in the behavior of individual organization members, but more often it is a characteristic of groups such as departments, power coalitions, administrative teams, and the like. [2] In all cases, resistance reflects a mixture of self-interest coupled with opinions, valid or invalid, as to what is good for the organization.

An individual alone can seldom mount strong resistance to major change, for he lacks power and will be perceived to be dominated by his own self-interest. The power of the individual roughly corresponds to his level in the hierarchy and to his control of strategic processes or resources. Although rank-and-file workers were not interviewed in this study, it can be said that in the absence of a labor union, their best means of resistance is to garner the support of other individuals and groups. Since the powers of the rank-and-file are limited, overt resistance is minimized, and resistance is driven beneath the surface or transferred to forms of dissatisfaction more likely to receive attention.

According to Victory's chaplain, people resist change "as a matter of conserving energy. There are always emotional costs in change, so many will resist." Yet people do learn to accept change. One of the laboratory managers stated that:

> I've learned a lot here. I've learned to change and to
> accept change. I never thought I could. I never used
> to be that way at all. In fact, they used to say about
> me that if I were here at the beginning, we'd still be
> running on square wheels.

Let us now examine resistance to change as it was found in Victory Hospital internally to an organizational unit, between one or more units, and among members of occupational groups, such as nurses, physicians, and technicians.

RESISTANCE TO INTERNAL CHANGE

Changes internal to a unit, that is, with few or no effects on other units, were among the simplest to implement. Here the principal approach involved strong supervisory management. For example, with respect to the new patient profile system inaugurated by the pharmacy, according to the chief pharmacist:

Our drug distribution remained the same. Also, we
didn't have to change any of the forms that the doctors
use in making out the patient medicine request; therefore, they weren't really aware we had made a change.
Most of the effects of the new system were centered
right here in the pharmacy, in that we had to implement a new night courier position and a full-time
secretarial position plus two profile clerks.

And in the medical records department, according to the director:

I doubt if there are any direct effects that our innovations have on other departments. However, I believe
there are indirect effects. From our automated system, I've been able to generate several types of data
and break them down into several categories useful to
department heads and some people on the higher administration level in controlling their departments.
. . . Mostly, however, the data that I generate is
used right here in the department. I felt that the activity report was needed to give a visual picture of
the department and to justify our manpower requirements. Also, by looking at this data I can tell who in
the department is doing the least work. In other
words, I can monitor what the output of my people is.

Internal change and resistance to it were most evident in the
nursing services department headed by the vice president, Winters.
Most of these changes were adopted only after extensive study of
costs, patient benefits, or advantages to nurses. Yet the strong ad-
vocacy of the vice president was everywhere apparent. On occasions
when subordinate groups could vote on a change, an undercurrent of
resistance continued even after a vote favoring continuance or adoption. An example is provided by events associated with the implementing of team nursing. The assistant director of nursing indicated
some of the advantages, but also stressed the difficulties:

The team system is good. People assigned to a team
generally stay in one particular wing, so problems do
develop. They do get to know their patients, so in
that sense it approximates the primary care system.
But people get into their habits and routines, so sometimes we lose flexibility. It is hard to adjust to ill-
nesses and absentees, for example. When we have to
change people from one team to another, they don't

like it very much. Some people like change and some
don't. To some it is an adventure and to others it is
a threat.

Another difficulty that came to light during the implementation
stage was that physicians could not or would not readily identify the
appropriate team leader for the particular wing where their patients
were located:

> Interviewer: . . . the nurses from the different teams
> are all in the central core area?
> Assistant Director of Nursing: Yes, that's right, and
> the doctors don't always recognize which nurse
> goes with which wing. They don't take the time,
> although if they did look at the wall charts, they
> would know. But you can't get the doctors to do
> that. Now it might be true that the nurse doesn't
> know the answer to the doctor's questions but she
> shouldn't say "that's not my job." She should tell
> him she'll help him find out.

In spite of such difficulties, there were few if any serious expectations of eliminating the team concept in favor of primary nursing. A major factor blocking this reversal was the probable need to
increase the number of RNs and LPNs and to reduce the number of
nursing assistants, thereby increasing operating costs:

> Interviewer: So you don't think you will go back to
> primary nursing?
> Assistant Director of Nursing: Well, I can't predict
> what will happen. Staffing problems will play a
> big part in such a decision. We really couldn't go
> back to primary nursing on a 24-hour-a-day
> basis. . . . So the advantage of teams is that
> we use fewer RNs. It's a great manpower saving,
> and in order to return to primary nursing we
> would have to be assured of getting enough pro-
> fessional help.

Nevertheless, the return to primary nursing care remained a
fervent hope on some of the patient care floors. According to one
of the unit coordinators, the hiring of more RNs and LPNs would
make this possible:

Interviewer: What kind of plan do you have that
brings all the things that you want to do together?
Unit Coordinator: First of all, we are going to hire
more registered nurses and licensed practical
nurses and start phasing out the nursing assistants.
Hopefully, this will lead to primary nursing, that
is, each nurse taking care of a given number of
people instead of being a member of a team. Right
now there are two units in the hospital making a
pilot study of primary nursing. It has been approved by the nursing staff and now awaits approval
from administration. The reason we are having to
go through the bureaucratic processes is that it is
going to cost more money. We are going to have
to hire more professionals.

The views of the vice president and the assistant director of
nursing appeared to be ambivalent. Team nursing has been favored
by the National Nursing Association; since there were mixed feelings
on the nursing floors, continuance of the team system could be predicted for quite some time:

Interviewer: Do you think primary nursing might
come back?
Assistant Director of Nursing: Not according to what
I found out at the meeting in San Francisco. . . .
There's so much to know. It's very complex and
there's a lot of details to study. At the meeting
we divided into groups and there was a team RN
person to visit all the groups to talk about it.
However, it turned out that she didn't know much
and we didn't find out anything we didn't know
already.

The nursing department experienced resistance in a number
of other internal matters. A key factor in changes in the nursing
department was the strong supervision of Winters. She verbalized
the importance of participation and involvement as routes to change,
yet was perceived by persons inside and outside the department as
heavy-handed and autocratic. Winters herself stated that:

It makes a difference what group you are talking about.
Our unit coordinators are very receptive to change.
For example, if our method of assigning patients is
right or wrong that's something I can get them to

consider and if we need a change, it can be worked out. But you can't change people by just telling them to change.

Yet the chaplain, an external observer, reported a different view:

There's a problem in nursing. The unit coordinators feel that they have no part in effective change. Change is from the top down. Now this isn't any one person's fault. It's something like a religious order. It's hard to get participation and to get the negative feedback that is needed. Suppose some people feel that an idea should be put on the shelf. There's a lot of indifference in Victory but at least resisters help us take account of negative feedback. We need that. Some people feel threatened and others don't.

An example of the use of strong decision making to reinforce change, in this instance, increasing work loads among nurses, was Winters's action on nursing histories. According to the evening house supervisor, the task of taking nursing histories had been delegated to the nursing assistants. When Winters decided this was ineffective, she gave orders that the RNs would henceforth do them. The RNs complied, but complained about the added burden.

Despite her authoritarianism, Winters did experience a failure of innovation which caused her to acknowledge the limitations of administrative fiat:

When I first came here I was very naive about management. . . . I got an idea once from a salesman, who was selling . . . some beautiful boards for scheduling people's time. I thought it was a great idea so I bought everybody one of these boards. We spent over $1,000 on them. And they are down in the storeroom now. Nobody would use them. When I first gave them their boards I almost got run off the premises. They wouldn't even watch me demonstrate it. So you see, the people in an organization have thought about problems I never would think of. . . .

Resistance in nursing was frequently encountered in the reassignment of nurses from one floor to another. According to the assistant director for staff education, this was largely due to failure to explain the changes in advance to the persons affected:

I feel that this hospital, any hospital really, is extremely subject to change, and while people are resistant to it in some respects, it almost becomes a way of life in others. For example, pediatrics recently moved from the first to the eighth floor and in effect we had to reassign some personnel. Therefore there were personal adjustments to be made. There was resistance by the people who were already occupying the eighth floor because they had not adequately prepared for the change. That is, when the new people arrived on the eighth floor they were like strangers taking over. I think sometimes we forget that other people have feelings too. We move so fast sometimes that we forget about interpersonal relationships.

In nursing there was extensive resistance to projects initiated by the assistant directors of nursing and for staff education and the assistant director for specialized personnel and special studies. Problems of implementation developed around the mechanics of carrying out new programs. New staff education programs provide an example. According to the assistant director:

We have some problems of implementation. One of the main ones is scheduling hours for classes so that they don't interfere with patient coverage. We usually handle this by having classes staggered, so there is always someone who can cover for someone else. Another problem we usually face . . . is that of wisely using the time we have available. We usually have to decide what to zero in on to make the teaching program effective.

The staff education unit failed to implement successfully a new program of group meetings designed to improve internal communications:

Interviewer: Can you think of an innovation or change that has been unsuccessful in nursing?
Assistant Director: I can think of a problem that is directly concerned with communications and the fact that people are not very well informed around here. In the light of this problem, staff education came up with a plan whereby we would communicate with the staff through groups which

would have elected leaders and people would be assigned to these groups. There was an unbelievable amount of paperwork involved and the final result was that these planned monthly meetings never did go very well. After one or two of them, we decided to just give up. We figured it was for the benefit of the employees and if they didn't want it, why should be bother?

Interviewer: Was it ever determined why the new system didn't work?

Assistant Director: No. I believe everyone lost interest but we did send out memos and so forth. Certain individuals, the group leaders, that is, were given the responsibility of making sure that these group sessions were communicated, that everyone knew about them who was supposed to. There was just really general apathy.

Interviewer: That's very interesting.

Assistant Director: Isn't it though! Mrs. Winters got the idea when she visited another hospital that had worked out this group type of communication. She said that it had worked beautifully, but it just hasn't worked here. It could have been because management consultants had administered the communications program in other hospitals. Prior to this group approach, I had tried to initiate monthly staff nurse meetings but they haven't come off either. Recently, Mrs. Winters's office and staff education have been pushing for Mr. Wright to get the same consultants to come here and implement the group program.

Getting nurses to accept responsibilities for patient education also proved difficult for nursing's staff education unit. One of the coordinators indicated that the resistance related to the additional work and doubts about nurses having the right skills:

Interviewer: How does the nursing staff feel about the prospect of having to take on this additional responsibility of patient education?

Unit Coordinator: . . . it should be one of our primary functions. I would say about 50 percent of the nursing staff on the eleventh floor like the idea and think it would be an interesting thing to learn how to do this. The other half is not very enthusiastic.

Interviewer: Why aren't they enthusiastic?
Unit Coordinator: Well, I feel that they're afraid
to try it because they don't know how to teach
and see themselves as already having plenty of
work to do.

The pressures of resistance were also keenly felt by the assistant director for specialized personnel and special studies. Resistance was generated by the need for the staff unit to multiply its efforts by teaching the nurses to teach, thereby increasing their duties:

This is where our specialized personnel come in not
only to take on the responsibility of patient education
but to teach nurses how to teach patients. It's practically impossible to assume, for instance, that one
cardiovascular specialist can teach all of the cardiovascular patients in the hospital how to take care of
themselves and what they should know. Therefore it
seems only reasonable that nursing should take on
this added responsibility. Of course, Mrs. Winters
feels this way also, yet it's quite another thing to get
unit coordinators and staff nursing to become involved
and start doing patient education on a regular basis.
We've met a lot of resistance in this area.

The staff specialists often found that resistance to change could lead to conflict. The following account of a classical case of line-staff conflict came from the assistant director for specialized personnel in nursing:

I have experienced a lot of jealousy and envy toward
specialized personnel from the nursing staff, primarily because we don't have to work weekends and
we have flexible schedules. We work independently
and in general we are thought of as the fair-haired
children of Mrs. Winters. These attitudes don't
help our specialists . . . and they contribute to the
resentment which is manifested in resistance to new
ideas that specialists propose. . . . These specialists have formed a group called the Nursing Specialists Council. It was formed before I became assistant director and it functions in implementing new
policies within the nursing organization. Both the
nursing specialists and Mrs. Winters feel that it is

nursing's responsibility to teach patients. Therefore, the specialists work together to convince
nurses, through the chain of command, that this is
what they should be doing and tell them how they
should do it. . . . When our plans of action are
ready, the four specialized nurses will present them
to each unit coordinator meeting. . . . Most of the
time they seem receptive, yet things just do not get
implemented like they should. The specialized personnel can't go directly to a staff nurse on a nursing
wing and tell her what to do and how to do it unless
she asks, simply because they don't have authority
or responsibility. We have to go through the chain
of command and therefore accountability for these
plans . . . becomes a problem. The specialized
personnel try to be as helpful as possible.

RESISTANCE TO CHANGES INVOLVING
MULTIPLE UNITS

Whereas both strong supervision and highly participative management styles can be instrumental in change internal to a unit,
changes having impacts on other units require higher-level coordinating decisions and different forms of persuasion and cooperation. Administrative units become self-protective domains which value autonomy, cohesion, and solidarity of purpose around a central mission.
This often leads to conflict arising from defensive self-preservation.
The conflict becomes manifest either in blocking or preventing change
proposals or in slowing or killing changes after adoption.

On relatively simple issues, the parties in potential or actual
conflict often come to working understandings that mitigate or mediate the conflict. Trade-offs are allowed in which the parties say,
"You can change this if you'll let me change that." On more complicated issues, battle lines are drawn and higher coordinators are
put to the test.

Since nursing services are so pervasive in the operation of a
hospital, nursing was observed to be forced rather frequently into
changes necessitated by changes in other units. Accordingly, acceptance by nurses was important to the successful implementation
of many changes originating in other units. In such changes, acceptance generally stemmed from persuasion based on time saving
for nurses or on their potential for making the work of nurses easier.

Pharmacy provides an example of a unit where change has substantial impacts on nursing practice. Even where a change had

clear advantages for the nurses, however, change agents in the
pharmacy had to exercise a great degree of persuasion and pay
special attention to demonstrating its merits. Two changes were
successfully implemented in this way: the new patient profile system and the change to 24-hour-a-day availability of a registered
pharmacist to dispense medications from the pharmacy. One of the
pharmacists indicated that selling the advantages (relieving evening
and night shift nurses from finding a key and obtaining their own
medications) reduced the resistance, but in the case of the 24-hour
availability of a pharmacist, a more elaborate persuasion effort
was necessary. He sold the change as a morale booster:

> Interviewer: What indication did you have that it was
> a morale booster?
> Chief Pharmacist: Before I implemented the plan, I
> went to a monthly meeting of the supervisory
> nurses and told them that we were ready to go
> ahead, and explained more fully what would be in-
> volved. They really appreciated what I had done,
> and, as a matter of fact, signed a letter of appre-
> ciation and sent it to me personally. I can under-
> stand why they like the idea of not having all that
> responsibility. A lot of drugs here in the pharmacy
> have to be accounted for daily and most of them are
> lethal in some way. At any rate, the new system
> took pressure off the coordinators and gave them
> more time to concern themselves with their admin-
> istrative and medical responsibilities.
> Interviewer: Was there any group that you know of,
> say, for instance, LPNs or orderlies, that re-
> sisted this new idea?
> Chief Pharmacist: I can't recall one single person
> that resisted this new system. It may have meant
> more work for the unit clerks administratively,
> but it really made the system easier to work with
> for everyone concerned. We virtually had no prob-
> lems with the new system except maybe for staff-
> ing. . . . It takes a special kind of person to want
> to work nights. We had a lot of people in our de-
> partment try it but they didn't like it. Now, how-
> ever, we have a very stable staff.

Two other changes in the pharmacy, however, aroused nursing's strong resistance to change: the introduction of the intravenous
medication program and the institution of the Brewer medication

system. Within the pharmacy, however, there was disagreement over the predictions of resistance or acceptance. One of the pharmacists, for example, felt that the new IV plan would be accepted merely by persuading nurses and doing research on its objective merits:

> Interviewer: What sort of preparations do you think will have to be made before the new IV program can be implemented?
>
> Pharmacist: Well, for one thing, we are going to have to get some ideas on how to operate the program from hospitals that have already implemented it. I suppose this will involve quite a bit of travel. . . . After we formulate the plan, we are going to have to work with nursing and sell them on it. I don't believe this is going to be very difficult. We are also going to have to work out a procedure for filling orders. Also, somewhere along the line we are going to have to have some formal training for our pharmacists and maybe even hire another one.
>
> Interviewer: So you think that nursing is going to accept this new program wholeheartedly?
>
> Pharmacist: Yes, I think they will as a matter of fact, because this is going to mean less work for them. Because of tradition, I think there will probably be some resistance but in the end I think it will be accepted. I am personally going to push the program by emphasizing the advantage of sterility. I believe this is one of the big plus factors with the program.

However, the chief pharmacist had more reservations about the degree of nursing resistance to the new IV program:

> Interviewer: This is obviously a good thing for the patient. Why do the nurses persistently resist this program?
>
> Chief Pharmacist: Well, they have two standard arguments. One, the philosophy of the old school of nursing says don't administer any medicine that you don't mix yourself. Two, the nurses claim that this method of premixing the medicine wouldn't combine with their method of administering IVs, namely, the piggyback system.

Piggyback IVs are connected in a T-joint going into
one patient. The nurses claim that because of this
method of administering IVs, our IV additive program wouldn't be of any help.

Interviewer: Why do you think that administration
doesn't push for the implementation of the IV additive program? It seems like it would benefit the
patient.

Chief Pharmacist: That's a good question. I don't
push ideas around here. I sell ideas. After all,
it's the nurses who are going to have to make it
work. Without their voluntary wholehearted support, I don't think we can make any system work.

Ultimately the new IV system was adopted. There was resistance to the change, but at least one unit coordinator combated
the resistance by forceful administrative leadership, leaving nurses
no choice but to change:

I have many different approaches to leadership and I
was very autocratic in this case. I just told them
that they didn't have a choice, that quality of care was
the issue, and this was the way it was going to be done.
I knew there was resistance or friction, but I stressed
that we could do it. I told them that I knew they could
do it, that it was important and I wasn't going to listen
to any excuses.

Some problems of resistance endure for long periods of time.
The Brewer medication system requires the nurse to pour each
dose of medication at the time it is to be given to the patient instead of prepouring medications in advance. Although this system
was instituted several years prior to this study, it was still being
resisted at the time of interviewing in late 1974. According to the
evening house supervisor in nursing:

The nurses and aides still do it the way they want to.
I agree that that part of the Brewer medication system is impractical because it requires so much time
and effort by the nurse to pour for each patient individually. . . . Sometimes I get the distinct feeling
that the policy writers here in the executive offices
have never really administered to a patient because
of the discrepancy between the practical situation
and policy.

Increases in work and responsibility were factors in resistance to two other changes initiated externally but having an impact on nursing. One was in x-ray procedures and the other in procedures for handling specimens going to the laboratory. Both examples were reported by the evening house supervisor:

> Interviewer: How do innovations in other areas affect nursing service?
>
> House Supervisor: The effect is usually in the form of a greater demand made on us. . . . This demand is usually in the form of some increase in administrative duties. For example, not long ago we were told instead of sending two request forms down with every specimen that we not only label the tube that the specimen was in but we send three different-colored request forms down. I feel that if the lab needs all that information then they should do it instead of nursing.

And, on x-ray procedures:

> Sometimes I feel I can't support some of the things that are suggested simply because there are just too many ideas that cause frustration. For example, our administrative duties seem to increase whenever x-ray has some kind of change in their department. Not long ago we just had to fill out one x-ray request; now we have to fill out three. The same holds true for a lot of other interdepartmental activities. Another cause is the fact that Mrs. Winters is a perfectionist.

Changes by the various laboratories constituted another source of change required of nursing. In the radiology laboratory, for example, the laboratory staff failed to persuade nurses on the night shift to accept responsibility for locating someone to transport patients to the laboratory. The chief radiological technician went over the head of the vice president of nursing, taking the problem to higher administration. According to the chief:

> We have a problem of transportation after 9 p.m. It's hard to get patients except from the emergency room. The emergency room staff brings patients right in for us, but from the rest of the hospital we are supposed to get them. The nurses call and want the technicians

to come right up. The runners aren't on duty so the
technicians get the call. But we can't spare the
technicians. We can't have them running around
the hospital finding the patients. They have to stay
here to do the work. I was very sorry to have to
take this problem to higher administration.

The chief had suggested that the night house nursing supervisor
should be designated as the one responsible for finding a person to
transport patients to the laboratory:

The proposed solution would be a great help. We
always used to have full cooperation from the house
supervisor and I don't know what's gone wrong.
Suddenly it stopped. The thing is that the house
supervisor knows everything that's going on at night
in the hospital. She knows where people are likely
to be and would be able to find somebody that could
transport the patient for us. There isn't enough to
justify full-time people, and at that hour of the
night we just can't send our technicians out for the
patients.

RESISTANCE BY OCCUPATIONAL GROUPS

Each occupational group within the hospital has its cluster of
preferred values, beliefs, therapeutic protocols, habits, traditions,
aims, and organizational roles. These elements may individually
or collectively bear the impact of change efforts. That impact will
be a function of the individuals' commitments to the various elements, of the strength of the change attempts, and of the collective
strength the occupational group can assemble to preserve its fundamental tenets.

We have already seen in the preceding section that the nursing services staff in Victory viewed proposed changes in large part
according to what nursing in general ought to think. Physicians,
too, exhibited the same tendency. An illustration is provided by the
attempt nationally to train and employ physicians' assistants. Such
training programs have now been largely abandoned. In Victory,
the physician heading the anesthesiology group reported that there
was strong resistance to physicians' assistants largely because
nurses in anesthesiology are already present in the role of assistant
and there would be additional conflict for the physician to manage:

Interviewer: What is your opinion about the extent
of change and innovation going on in this hospital?
Physician: I would describe things here as being
revolutionary.
Interviewer: Could you give me an example?
Physician: Have you ever heard of our physicians'
assistant program? (Laughing) In the field of
anesthesiology we are beginning to use a few,
around the nation, that is. But we don't do it at
Victory. There is a move to do it here but I hope
it is aborted. There is a definite move to make
use of additional personnel to help the physicians,
like technologists and other types. And we already
have the help of the nurses in anesthetics. I don't
see any need for another group of assistants. The
problem is that all of the assistants must be under
the control of the anesthesiologist. If we have
assistants, we have the problem of conflicts with
the nurses, and it's a management problem for us
to avoid too much independence on the part of the
nurses. Fortunately here at Victory this is not a
serious problem because the nurse has no choice.
It is a select group. We get a lot of them from our
own school of nurse anesthetists. They are used to
working with physicians and they have had only physicians around when they need help during their
training.

Another example of direct physician resistance to administrative change was seen in the pathology laboratory. According to Vice
President Watson, who was acting in the role of change agent:

. . . not long ago I went to an American College of
Hospital Administrators meeting where we discussed
the merits and demerits of having a laboratory manager who is not a pathologist or a physician. This is
an idea we haven't been able to implement here. The
pathologist in charge won't change. She won't let anyone handle her administrative responsibilities and we
are still trying to persuade her. It would be such a
big help to her and to us.

Rightly or wrongly, the members of one occupational group
often attribute resistance to another group. The vice president of
nursing blamed physicians for the inability of Victory Hospital to
establish an outpatient program:

Vice President of Nursing: . . . we are facing the
   problem of what to do about outpatient needs. We
   don't do much of that here. I think we should bend
   to these pressures from the public and offer the
   services they want.
Interviewer: Why haven't you, then?
Vice President of Nursing: I think the doctors are the
   cause of it. The physicians will come here for an
   emergency and take somebody's appendix out, but
   they don't want to come here and treat anybody
   with a cold. They haven't interfered with our
   handling of emergencies, but they won't let us
   develop the outpatient care. We need a staff of
   doctors here 24 hours a day just to see sick people.

Clearly, resistance to change in hospitals such as Victory is
compounded of a number of complex factors reaching beyond the
hospital itself. As difficult as purely internal change may be, it is
even more difficult to institute change where resistance finds the
broad support of professional or technological views from outside.
The answers to the problem are to be found in administrative behavior designed to combat or prevent resistance. This will now be
analyzed in the final section of this chapter.

OVERCOMING RESISTANCE TO CHANGE

The foregoing descriptions of resistance to change contain a
number of implied strategies for minimizing or overcoming possible
or actual resistance. Among these are the use of positional authority and strong supervision to contain the opposition or obtain compliance, however grudging; and less coercive strategies centering
in the planning process, including the timeliness and appropriateness of change, and the use of participation and co-optation aimed
at involving those affected by the proposed changes.

During implementation, resistance often continues after formal acquiescence to a change. This postadoption resistance is a
residue of opposition which could not be overcome by earlier strategies followed in prior planning stages. It is met, however, chiefly
by continuing the early strategies of supervision, participation, involvement, and co-optation strengthened by a factor which may be
called persistence. The drive to persist emerges from the commitment by change agents or administrators—in which the endurance of
an adoption decision stems from the application of resources to the
change, the training of personnel, and the impact on the management
reputation of the proponents of change.

The causes of resistance are varied, and we have seen that they include characteristics of the individual, the constraints of organization, and the influences of external pressures from technical expertise, professionalism, or public demands. Change strategies, to be effective in reducing resistance, should bear a logical relationship to causation. Yet Victory's administrators were more pragmatic than analytical in selecting their strategies. They expected resistance and were aware of the need to come to grips with their own roles as change agents. But the primary method was to rely on authority or obvious merits to justify adoptions, with the result that efforts to overcome resistance came during the implementation stage. This permitted the change agents to employ strategies more directly targeted to the nature of the actual resistance and to minimize their efforts to forecast the nature of that resistance.

Whereas the strategies of using positional authority, participation, involvement, and co-optation, the stressing of economic or pecuniary advantages, and timely communication were primarily intended to bolster the adoption process, there were also a number of coping strategies designed to make the decision stick, to improve the effectiveness of changes, and to reduce the dissonance underlying resistance to changes. Both the adoption and the coping strategies were employed as needed, usually in combined ways depending on the feedback information received by administrators. We will now analyze the following coping strategies: letting the passage of time smooth the transitions; persistence in reinforcing, supporting, and renewing the change or change program; and some form of teaching or instruction to acquaint organization members with new practices or skills.

The following example shows how the manager of food services simultaneously used the strategies of time, co-optation, and strong supervision:

> . . . there's always a few people that don't want to go along with a change and they usually manifest their discontent verbally. However, some people are open-minded about change. For example, when I came here I made several changes in our cooking methods. One was to introduce what's called progressive cooking . . . cooking food as it is needed and not all in one batch. . . . Food should be cooked in small quantities to get the full nutritional quality and to make it taste better. . . . It was hard to get the cooks to change from the old system of cooking everything at one time to the progressive system, and I had to fire a few of them. After a while, though, most of them

came around and saw the wisdom of the concept and
were willing to go along with the program even though
it did mean a little more work. The way I usually
handle introducing new concepts is to take a lot of
small steps instead of one big change, and I feel if
you can get people to thinking along the same lines as
you are, you can actually lead them into believing it
was their idea and that way you can get a lot more
cooperation.

Letting time pass so that employees can get used to a change
was seldom utilized as a single strategy, because the administrator
or department head can readily use other strategies with it. Teaching and instruction require time, as do the effort to co-opt recalci-
trant individuals and the need to involve participants in ironing out
difficulties.

Even aggressive advocates of change, such as the vice president of nursing, recognized the multifaceted nature of resistance
and the need to cope with the change:

Being a teacher of nursing before I came here, I had
a lot of ideas from my teaching. I brought these ideas
with me and I thought everybody would lap them up . . .
but no, it didn't work that way. There was a great reluctance and I found out that I had to be very patient
and it took hard work to get changes made. We've
learned to politick a little. You have to plant seeds
now and then and let the seeds grow. I also think to
get change you have to get a discussion going and
listen to people.

Changes that were relatively invisible aroused little resistance. However, where there are major impacts on task performance, training designed to change work behavior and improve
motivation becomes important. In the new computerization program at Victory, both invisible and visible changes occurred. The
new personnel records system maintained at Norfield, for example,
had low visibility:

Interviewer: Did you encounter much resistance to
change on this project?
Acting Director of Personnel: No, we didn't and that
is a surprise. Actually I would have said to you
that 99.44 percent of the people are against any
kind of change, especially if they think it's going
to affect them in any way.

Interviewer: So you think that this change wasn't too
   visible to them?
Acting Director of Personnel: That's right. They
   couldn't care less because they don't see anything
   really happening. It's not too unusual and all they
   know is something's going on in the office. They
   can't see where it affects them very much so we
   didn't get any resistance to change.

Yet the change to a computerized records system in the business
office to improve billing and other business processes required
many job changes and was still incomplete after three years. According to a financial counselor, instructional classes, coupled with
the intrinsic motivation inherent in the new procedures, were important:

The two things that I was most aware of about the employees was their own curiosity and lack of knowledge.
The consultants had stimulated our interest in the new
system because they told us that after we learned how
to operate it properly it would save us a lot of time
and make our jobs easier. They conducted classes in
which they explained how to set up new accounts and
how changes had to be made in our old system to make
it mesh better with the computerized system. While
all these training sessions were being conducted by
the consultants, we in the business office set about to
create a hospital information profile . . . to contain
all the information necessary to carry a patient
through a hospital stay administratively. This is
where we made our first real mistake . . . because
we didn't look around at other hospitals and see what
information they had been using in this hospital profile. We just took a large amount of information and
figured that we would modify it as we went along and
in six months we would have information that we
needed. But it's been three years now and there's
still information that we don't have. . . .

Working with individuals who are willing to learn eases the
potential for resistance to change. For example, the supervisor of
the neurosciences laboratory reported that:

Occasionally a technician will get huffy when we have
to change a procedure. However, they know that the

change is for the best and they generally go along
with it. I feel that the technicians we have . . .
right now are fairly open when it comes to learning
new procedures. They are open mainly because the
doctors on the staff of this department and myself
have taught them what they know and they are confident we will teach them anything they should know or
will need to know in the future. This is a concern
when I think about the new technicians we will be
getting from the Technical Institute who will have
their knowledge obtained from another source and
may not be as open when it comes to learning. . . .

A combination of classroom, work experience, and involvement through feedback was used to help nurses change from glass
to electronic thermometers. According to the director of staff
education in nursing:

We've had enough experience to know that there's going to be resistance to new ideas and therefore we
must plan every change. A good example is when we
went from glass to electronic thermometers. Before
we attempted to implement the new system, we had
classes at all levels in the nursing organization.
This was intended as an orientation to the new procedures. . . . We explained why we were going to
use electronic thermometers and we explained the
correct procedure. We also gave the nurses practical instructions and let them try them under supervision. After we had done all this, including the
setting of a definite date for the implementation of
the change, we asked for feedback from the people
who had been attending the orientations. I feel that
feedback is important because people need the opportunity to express their feelings. I honestly believe that this recognition of feeling . . . is possibly
one of the most important stages in the implementing of change.

Sensitivity to potential communication problems that pervade
the hierarchical structure helps the change agent minimize resistance. For example, resistance to change in the maintenance department was encountered from rank-and-file employees as well
as from physicians, and sensitivity to levels in the chain of command was deemed important:

Interviewer: Do you experience resistance to ideas
that are generated here in your department? If
so, how do you handle this?

Director: Yes, quite often. I have to work with so
many people on so many different levels that one
of the basic challenges of my job is minimizing
this resistance. I have to work with people in
housekeeping who are not on the same level . . .
with the doctors, and I have to be able to communicate and get along with all of them. I have
to wear so many hats in my job that I'm really
kind of a salesman, I guess, in that there is a different approach to getting along with everyone. As
a specific example of resistance, I have here a
memo about a suggestion that Mr. Ellis wanted on
modifications for surgery. I made the recommen-
dation. However, I received resistance from some
of the doctors. . . . What it amounted to was that
the doctors wanted to discuss the modification
problem immediately and I didn't want to discuss
it with them because I always talk to Mr. Ellis
about things of this nature before I discuss it with
anyone outside my immediate chain of command.
This is not to say that I don't discuss some of my
functions and responsibilities with doctors. It's
just that in situations like this I like to inform my
boss first so that they won't short-circuit the
plan. . . .

Sensitivity to variations in skills or attitudes among different
age groups was found helpful in the physical therapy department.
Resistance was viewed as a dichotomy between older and newer employees, with the younger employees being less resistant to change.
Therefore the head of the department followed a strategy of hard-
line supervision coupled with efforts to improve interpersonal relations:

Interviewer: The changes that you've mentioned are
very interesting. Are you aware of resistance by
any of your physical therapists?

Department Head: Well, I'll have to answer that
question "yes." The older therapists, and we
have a couple of them on our staff, are more resistant to changing procedures and techniques than
the younger ones. I'm aware that some of our

therapists are waiting for retirement. However,
the younger ones are more willing to learn and are
more receptive to new ideas simply because they
know if they are going to work in this field they
will have to learn on a yearly, monthly, weekly,
and daily basis almost.

Interviewer: You've mentioned some personality conflict in your department. In spite of that, there's
no heavy resistance to change?

Department Head: No, I don't think resistance is
strong, not overt resistance anyhow. The group
of therapists I had before worked together a lot
better than the ones I have now. I didn't have to
supervise them or tell them what to do. If there
was a job to be done, they were willing to be there
and help or do it themselves. Communication and
general interpersonnel relations were also a lot
better. . . . However, if I have to act like a boss,
I will, and therefore, I'm firm with this group and
I make sure the work gets done.

Occasionally, an appeal to logic, self-interest, or patient
welfare was used to improve functions impeded by resistance. In
the new parent education program among OB-GYN nurses, resistance from both nurses and doctors appeared during implementation,
and it was combated by emphasizing life-saving benefits. According to a unit coordinator:

. . . most of the doctors objected to having fathers in
the delivery room because if they got sick it would be
one more problem to handle and it could put a serious
strain on . . . the personnel in the delivery room.
Another valid point was, how would anyone be able to
tell the father that he had to leave the delivery room
if some contingency arose? There is a question as
to whether the father could be objective if something
did happen. As far as the nurses were concerned,
specifically the two older nurses in the nursery,
their primary objective was to keep the babies secure,
and to keep a watch on them. Also, the nurses . . .
thought that there would be more work. . . . I had to
show the nurses that in the long run it would be less
work for them. The net result of the program has
been that things have improved.

In implementing the new medication nurse program, one of the unit supervisors indicated the hope that after the trials on her floor, the use of the idea would spread throughout the hospital. She found resistance low, having to co-opt only two resistant nurses. The example also illustrates how persistence in an effort pays off, since her first attempt to implement the program had failed, and only on the second attempt, after adjusting for suggestions from nurses, was the program successful.

The passage of time allows the objective merits of a change to become real to the persons affected, principally through concrete demonstrations of advantages to individuals. Acceptance of change is based on rational analysis. For example, a typist in the admitting department reported that:

> We've had quite a few changes since I came here, and as time goes on, it seems as though change becomes easier and easier to accept. I guess that's what it's all about though. One that was implemented when I first came here involved our switching to a color code for patients who had Medicare. If we started filling out one of these cards and a patient had forgotten a vital piece of information, such as he was on Medicare, we would have to start all over and lose quite a bit of time and energy. Therefore it was a desirable change. Everyone was for it and it was very readily accepted. . . . Another change involved the adoption of a modified patient information sheet. This was done because of computerization of the admitting system so that we needed less information. . . . We could store key data such as the price of the rooms . . . in the computer and could use codes to key the information in as we needed it. . . . Therefore, this meant less work for us. . . . Prior to the computerized system I had to figure out the times when the patients would move from one bed to another or from one service to another and this was really tedious. Now, however, all the scheduling is left to the computer and we have less chance for error this way.

Persistence in implementing change was further illustrated in the maintenance department, where a supervisory development program was interrupted by a strike which could have been used as an excuse to abandon the training. Instead, the head of this department said that "We are very optimistic and are going to keep pushing the program in the future." A supervisory training objective also was being implemented by the director of medical records, who found that on-the-job learning required a reversal of a previous decision change which put the supervisors in separate offices:

> The hardest thing I have done since I have been direc-
> tor is to try to implement a supervisory development
> program. . . . We have two graduates of medical
> record administration programs who are now first-
> line supervisors. . . . I've tried to give them pres-
> tige in putting them in the little closed-in office you
> saw when you came in. However, it didn't work.
> The employees kept coming to me with questions in-
> stead of to their immediate supervisors, and I ended
> up doing quite a bit of their work. I decided recently
> that the solution to the problem was to bring them out
> of that closed-in office and get them closer to the
> people that they were supervising. What they were
> doing was sitting in that little office all day abstract-
> ing and coding and not learning how to relate to
> people. After I moved them out of the office, I noted
> that they dealt with the employees and the employee
> problems as they arose differently than I did. Their
> philosophy was different. However, now that they are
> exposed to the employees more, they are beginning to
> come around. My philosophy is that if you hire a per-
> son to do a job, you ought to let him do it. Therefore
> I will teach a person as much as I can about how to do
> his job, but when I feel he's learned enough I'll leave
> him alone and let him do the job. The problem with
> my supervisors was that they just weren't learning.
> I'd like to think that those two supervisors would be-
> come so good that I'd not have to criticize them at all.

The value of persistence coupled with co-optation was also demonstrated in attempting to change one of the nursing floors from primarily a medical care floor to a medical-surgical floor. The unit coordinator had asked Winters to make the change, but after four months the floor was still receiving only medical patients. According to the unit coordinator, the change approved by Winters was not implemented in the admitting office. She therefore first tried an indirect approach. When this failed, she took a direct approach with the director of admitting:

> Three or four months after I took the job . . . we
> were still getting nothing but medical cases up here.
> I went to Mrs. Winters and she told me that it had
> been changed. It was just that admitting was not send-
> ing the surgical patients to the floor. I figured the
> best thing to do was to go to admissions and remind
> them that we were a medical-surgical floor and that we
> could take surgical patients. I figured before I went
> storming in there and talked to the director I had bet-
> ter make a few friends in admissions first. So I
> would meet admitting people at lunch in the cafeteria
> and make friends with them and tell them that we
> wanted some surgical patients. This didn't really get
> any results, although I did make a lot of friends.
> When the time was right, I walked into the director's
> office and . . . reminded her that we were supposed
> to be a surgical floor and we would sure like to get
> some surgical patients. I told her that if there was
> any problem with the doctors or anyone else to let me
> know and I would help her out. But she assured me
> that there wasn't, and when I had gained her confi-
> dence and told her that we had a morale problem and
> reminded her of it a couple of times, she started send-
> ing surgical patients to the floor.

Earning confidence on the part of a change agent was an important consideration in many situations as a precondition for the
use of other strategies. For example, the director of the cardiovascular laboratory was perceived by some colleagues and superiors
to be a somewhat difficult person to work with. He himself recognized this, along with the need to develop his own interpersonal relationships:

> Interviewer: Your unit crosses a lot of organizational
> boundaries. Do you experience any resistance to
> change in the type of work you do?
> Director: Well, I came here in 1968 and I categorized
> Victory as being a tight hospital in that most of the
> RNs and most of the nurses that work here graduated
> from our own nursing school. I think I went two
> months before anyone spoke to me. However, my
> philosophy is that you never tell a person what you
> know; you show them. Since I considered the silent
> treatment I was getting as a personality problem, I
> knew it was just a matter of time before I overcame

it. Pretty soon the nursing staff, doctors, and the others began to realize that I was competent and I was accepted. The minimum amount of resistance that we've experienced here is in the OR where we have the most responsibility. We have no pump operators, per se. We have no standard procedures. Our objective is to maintain the patient hemodynamically and physiologically, all this of course under the direction of the doctor. I don't really have an opportunity to think about it too much because I am so busy but maybe the organization and my unit are too loose. But whatever, it seems to work extremely well.

In nursing, the unit coordinator system encountered resistances after organizational changes had been made. One problem, for example, was the articulation between the unit coordinator and the evening house supervisor. According to the supervisor:

Not long ago the nursing offices were decentralized and the linking pattern type of organization structure was implemented. This type of structure was set up to use unit coordinators who were directly responsible for 24-hour coverage on the units. The main problem is that they are not directly responsible to me, yet I have the responsibility for all the nursing personnel and services throughout the hospital during my shift. This situation sometimes makes for conflict when I have to pull personnel from an adequately staffed unit such as the fourth floor and place them in units where they are needed more.

Winters, the vice president of nursing, persisted in the implementation of the unit coordinator system, using a coping strategy of seeking a vote of affirmation from the nurses:

I'm very much aware of the innovation and creativity that is going on, but it is resisted, I'll have to say that. For example, when we established the unit coordinator system, a lot of the people were not sure of it. They complained a lot and they held back and they said they couldn't do things. So I went to them and said, "We're going to put this system to a vote and if you want it, fine, you'll have to say so and if you don't want it, we'll go back to the old system."

Of course it was all political. All unit coordinators
had a week to think it over and then we took their
vote. They wanted heavy responsibility and they
asked for the unit coordinator system to be maintained and that was the end of the complaining.

As noted earlier, strong supervision was found to be used
frequently in the implementation of change and in overcoming resistance. However, while this strategy was often successful internally, it often foreshadowed difficulties in the spread of an idea
to other units. In implementing the new intravenous medication
procedures, for example, backsliding was curbed but resistance
continued in other units:

Interviewer: Were there any instances of backsliding
into the old method?
Unit Coordinator: Yes, there were a couple of instances where there was some backsliding but I
told everyone that the next person I found that
didn't make the marks on the bottle and didn't do
it the way they were supposed to would be put on
report. This helped to get the point across that I
would accept nothing less than the standards that
had been set. When we had the system implemented
and running smoothly, I presented my results at a
meeting of all the nursing supervisors and they
seemed very receptive and said they liked it. As a
matter of fact, most of them were anxious to implement a similar system. At least that is what
they told me, but they never did it. I was rather
disappointed and felt that their defeatist attitude
was unjustified and if they had really tried they
could have done it because I showed that we could
do it and we are a fairly large unit up here on this
floor.

Failures to implement change sometimes occurred despite
strategies of strong supervision. When employees simply refuse
to act in accordance with the change, it is likely that the old methods
will prevail. One of the evening house supervisors indicated two
examples, one of them the ban against prepouring medicines under
the Brewer system and the other the failure of group meetings in
nursing:

Interviewer: What steps have been taken to imple-
    ment this portion of the Brewer medication sys-
    tem policy?
Supervisor: Usually, we'll get the word from Mrs.
    Winters that the old method has to stop and we've
    got to implement the new method and for one or
    two days we will, but sooner or later individuals
    will stop pouring the medicine as they administer
    and go back to prepouring. I'll tell you quite can-
    didly I don't try to enforce that policy because I
    think it's impractical.

And concerning the group meetings, according to the evening house
supervisor:

I have tried once-a-week meetings to work out our
problems, but they have been fairly ineffective. It's
not that they weren't well attended because they were,
but the main problem was that only petty problems
were discussed, the type that really there's no reso-
lution of and it usually turned into a gripe session.
Therefore, the meetings kind of fell by the wayside.

Another failure in change occurred in the attempt to implement a suggestion box system for employees. Here the issue was
also a lack of participation. According to the manager of food services:

I don't believe they have one now. However, just a
few years ago they had one, but it just seemed to
die. I don't think the employees got any kind of positive feedback, or felt like they were involved.

Teaching new methods was not always a guarantee of success.
This is illustrated by the new position of monitoring technician. It
was tried once, only to fail, but under a persistence strategy
coupled with instructional efforts, the assistant director for special
areas in nursing hoped ultimately to be able to make the plan work:

We are trying something new . . . called the monitoring technician. The monitoring technician watches the
oscilloscopes that are monitoring the heart rhythms of
patients in the unit. If we feel that we are successful
with this monitoring technician, we are going to extend
it to the medical intensive care unit and to the fifth

floor. We are hoping that this will free our nurses
for more patient care. It's very boring work for
nurses and because of this can be a source of
trouble. . . . Before I was first put in charge of
this area we had tried the monitoring technician program before and it didn't work. I can't really tell
you why, but we have taken individuals with little or
no background in hospital work and the cardiologist
has attempted to teach them some things about
rhythms. Now we are hoping it will work.

The success of a new program depends heavily on the abilities of supervisors and managers to show that monetary benefits
can be derived from the change. For example, the coordinator of
data control instituted a training program to combat problems with
patient charges:

The departments realized that they needed this program because they were losing money and also they
were having to do a lot of extra work because we
would send it back to them when it wasn't done properly. We also implemented a new charge system in
January and everyone was very cooperative. The
only complaint that I got was that we implemented it
too soon, the bugs weren't worked out of it. The
reason that everyone ultimately cooperated on the
new charge system was because I had personalized
the incentives. That is, I told them by not making
as much money for the department as they could they
were limiting their possibilities for pay raises. I
felt that this incentive plus the fact that our department tries to listen and develop a rapport was a tre-
mendous aid in implementing the new system.

Time allows persons affected by a change to gain firsthand
experience with its benefits. For example, the transcriber incentive pay program, one of the most successful innovations at Victory, was instituted because the transcribers had been too far behind the dictation and the work piled up. Vice President Watson
indicated that:

Our problem was that we just weren't getting the
amount of work out of the group that we thought it
was capable of producing. Also, it can be kind of
a routine and uninteresting job. Therefore, we

decided to pay an incentive amount above 500 lines a
day. At first there was a great deal of resistance
from the typists. They didn't understand what we
were trying to do and they were afraid of the change.
However, something like this works out if you allow
enough time. People get used to it and they come to
accept it better. Five years later now, you can't
take the system away from these people, they like it
so well.

Yet similar incentive programs had been planned for the
housekeeping and dietary departments, with no success:

Watson: We tried something similar in housekeeping,
but we finally had to drop the incentive. It just
didn't work. We also thought of trying it in the
dietary units, but it's awfully hard to get standards
and we haven't been able to do it there.
Interviewer: In the new transcriber incentive program,
do people complain because they might have better
tools or equipment than others?
Watson: No, the machines are all new and everybody
has the same equipment.
Interviewer: Did this program lead to any jealousies
or frustrations among the transcribers?
Watson: No, not really. The main objections came
from older people who couldn't make beyond the
standards.

Very few of the people interviewed at Victory expressed a
personal fear of change, although many managers felt that their
employees resisted change through fear of the unknown. The following statement by one of the admitting typists indicates how fear
of the unknown might build up as a precursor of resisting change
when supervisors fail to explain, teach, or communicate:

Not long ago I found out that the director was having
one of the night clerks count how many patients were
being admitted a day. She never said anything offi-
cially about what she was trying to do but I resent
whatever it is she is doing. I feel that because we
are working with individuals, and each person is different, it's difficult to set standards on how many
patients you should or should not admit per day. I
think it's unfair if any sanctions were to be imposed

on us because of these measurements and as I said,
I resent it now.

The same typist indicated the feeling that there was inadequate
involvement and participation in the admitting department:

> I feel that our director is a good person and a good
> supervisor but I also feel that most of the ideas she
> comes up with for the department are hers, not ours.
> It's not that anyone seems to mind very much that we
> don't have input into the system, it's just that it seems
> as though she listens but doesn't hear. We lean on her,
> though. None of us want her job because she works so
> hard. Most of the time I believe changes come about
> in this department by means of a letter from adminis-
> tration which the director will post on the department
> bulletin board and everyone is supposed to read and
> implement. Some changes, however, seem like wind
> in the air until we get word from administration.

To the extent that change agents and the implementers of
change are aware of individual attitudes and the need for communication, resistance can be minimized. The five strategies of strong
supervision, a participative approach, persistence, the passage of
time, and the use of teaching and instruction can do much to allevi-
ate the stress of change.

NOTES

1. Herbert Kaufman, The Limits of Organizational Change
(University: University of Alabama Press, 1971), pp. 5-40.
2. See, for example, the June 1979 issue of Nursing Dimensions, which is a theme issue on "Power in Nursing," edited by
D. E. McFarland and Nola Shiflett.

12

THE MANAGEMENT OF
INNOVATION AND CHANGE
IN HOSPITAL ORGANIZATIONS

In a hospital, as in any organization, the processes of managerial innovation and change derive from an intricate pattern of internal and external pressures. Since the hospital plays a critical role in our health care system, its capability for change and innovation is a matter of great importance. The external imperatives of change—society's demands for reducing costs, expanding services, and improving patient care—provide goals for the direction of change in the hospital, but the pace and extent of that change depend on the quality of managerial decision and action.

This study has focused on the need to understand how administrative behavior influences the processes of innovation and change in the hospital organization. The findings have been presented in the context of a feedback process model which departs from the commonly used linear sequence model. The feedback model portrays the basic elements of the organizational and managerial systems through which change occurs, and shows how these elements relate to the total process.

We can now bring together a number of conclusions and observations based on the findings of this exploratory study. They will emphasize practical strategies in terms of the following three topics: bureaucratic advantages and constraints, the role of technological change, and the need for a proactive strategy of change and innovation.

THE BUREAUCRATIC CONTEXT

Whether bureaucratic elements in an organization facilitate or inhibit change depends heavily on the ability of change agents to utilize bureaucracy's advantages and to combat its constraints.

Each hospital organization poses unique circumstances, but the consistencies which identify an organization as a bureaucracy reveal strengths and limitations that either block or facilitate change. To be an effective change agent, the individual is often in an adversary relationship to the system if not to particular superiors or colleagues. The unwary or unskilled change agent becomes discouraged and frustrated. The Machiavellian, authoritarian, or behaviorally unsophisticated change agent can make adoptions by positional authority, but risks frustration and failure in the implementation stages of change.

It is natural for those who desire change to blame the bureaucracy if they fail, or to congratulate themselves for overcoming it if they succeed. Whatever works in a bureaucracy can be deemed a success by bureaucrats. Given a sufficient amount of organizational slack, the bureaucracy can make even a clear-cut failure look like a valiant and magnificent try.

Victory's administrators held clear images of their successes and failures, despite the absence of concrete criteria for evaluation. While many changes occurred in Victory, few were truly innovative or significant breakthroughs in hospital administration or for our health care system. Instead, they were technical, mechanical, or procedural. Adoptions were based on economic criteria, and the human relations problems that followed adoption were met by expedients and adjustments, or a return to the status quo. Thus, Victory functioned satisfactorily at a maintenance level of change, but manifested few innovative changes of the type that seem to be called for by the public clamor for better and cheaper hospital and health care services.

This situation was partly due to a less than adequate understanding of the total change process depicted in the feedback model. Changes were considered mainly on an ad hoc and individual basis, rather than in relation to one another. Overall, comprehensive strategic planning for developmental change was not observed at Victory. Ad hoc change is logical in the bureaucratic context where change is directed according to the dictates of the bureaucracy's needs for survival, maintenance, or even gradual improvement.

Bureaucratic organizations possess a number of advantages for change within the above limitations. It is not widely perceived, for example, that bureaucracy often protects the would-be innovator. The element of risk to innovators and change agents in Victory was minimal, since there were no reprisals for attempts that did not succeed. Moreover, screening procedures deriving from bureaucratic precepts were so numerous and exacting that adopted ideas came to possess a rationale and a history that diffused both credit or blame beyond any single individual.

Another element of support for innovation and change in a bureaucracy is that of reference groups. Reference-group behavior was strong in Victory Hospital both internally and externally. The intense group consciousness among laboratory technicians, nurses, physicians, and other units undergirds change efforts by authenticating needs, providing sanctions and endorsements, and adding to efforts to persuade. The change agent need not, indeed usually cannot, act alone. Internal cohesion of a group, plus its affiliation with an outside association, provides a powerful support base for change internal to a unit. For example, the head of a laboratory may argue for a change "to get accreditation," or "to meet professional standards," or "to keep up with new thinking in our field." It also strengthens the case of a unit whose change proposals affect other units.

A real or an alleged crisis is often effective in producing bureaucratic change. Many organizations will not adopt a major innovation unless there is a crisis—an extreme change in conditions for which there is no adequate, programmed response.[1] The bureaucracy is organized to handle programmed responses and repetitive routines, and so is likely to avoid disruption of the status quo if at all possible. This accounts for the elaborate screening and evaluative procedures followed at Victory Hospital. Also relevant is a paradox first elucidated by Wilson: the factors that increase the probability that organization members will devise and present innovation proposals are precisely those factors that decrease the probability that the organization will adopt the proposals. This implies that the stimulation of potential innovations is distinct from, even antagonistic to, securing the adoption of innovations. He hypothesizes that the greater the diversity of an organization, the greater the probability that (1) members will conceive of major innovations, (2) major innovations will be proposed, and (3) the smaller the proportion of major innovative proposals that will be adopted.[2] This paradox seems particularly appropriate for Victory and the multi-unit organization type to which it belongs. Major innovations were few in number; major changes originated in events over which the hospital had relatively little control, such as the resignations of its top managers or the advancing technology in radiology.

Thus, it is a problem for today's hospital to bring about unusual and far-reaching innovations. But even if the hospital succeeds, there is a further problem of knowing what to do about an event of extraordinary innovation not previously covered by policy. Tradition and habit are the foes of change, but major changes requiring unique and far-reaching decisions force the organization to address itself to new needs. An organization's effectiveness in administering a stable system is not likely to transfer to the handling of large, unique, and new experiences. Growth in size also brings a firming up of bureaucratic elements, along with greater complexity. As an organization's maintenance behavior is institutionalized or routinized, it becomes more difficult to make significant innovations and changes.

Another feature of the bureaucratic organization that stifles innovation is fear reflected in the need to remain invisible. Thus, the fear of innovation goes with the bureaucratic life style. Common wisdom, for example, advises soldiers to "never be the first to do anything." This attitude produces the self-protective cover-ups which thwart innovation. Administrators can stifle innovation merely by arranging a paper-shuffling system. They pass ideas along to others, keeping copies of the memos for self-protection. Paper work advocating change is bounced up, down, and across the organizational network, where it often gets lost. Administrators can keep returning change proposals to their originators for minor corrections, or impose procedural blocks. They can use delay tactics, such as inept or powerless committees. A real expert at this can delay an idea for months, with a high probability that it will be forgotten or die a slow death.

Probably one of the greatest drawbacks to innovative behavior in bureaucratically organized hospitals lies in the nature of their reward systems. Despite the presence of organizational slack, Victory was unable specifically to reward innovative behavior. Nor did it disreward uncreative, noninnovative behavior. Its monetary reward system was geared to market rates; promotion opportunities were relatively limited. Thus, it relied on psychic or intrinsic rewards for innovation. Yet, innovations and changes often resulted in more—not less—work for those affected. Without tangible rewards, the incentive for change was low.

The inhibitive mechanisms of a bureaucracy are so extensive that an innovation defined as a successful change is a rare occurrence. It is really a lucky shot in the dark.[3] Moreover, the efficiency drive of the bureaucracy produces the opposite of conditions conducive to innovation. Earlier tenets of the "scientific management" mystique, which posit a system rooted in economic rationality, with efficiency the single, overarching organizational goal, are now transformed into management science: planning-programming-budgeting methods of control, applied mathematics, statistics, computers, rigorous measurement, and operations research methods for decision making and information processing.[4] But the constraining influences of bureaucracy remain, or even increase.

Similarly, the field of human relations has been transformed into an expanded discipline called organizational behavior. Whereas human relations attempted to ease the lot of humans in the bureau-cracy through improved management styles, organizational behavior concepts seek to change the bureaucracy itself in drastic ways, both as to structure and management style. At present, these sweeping changes have made no progress in hospital bureaucracies.

What is needed for innovation in hospitals is flexibility, plu-ralism, multiple approaches—exactly what efficiency experts decry as duplication or overlapping, and precisely what is offered by the open-system approach. This new form requires that all forms of suppression be ruled out. Competitive suspicion, distrust, and secrecy are replaced by mutual trust. Domains of knowledge re-place domains of power and authority. Rigid rules, such as "going through channels," are no longer important. Instead, new knowledge, ideas, and innovative changes would be openly and freely commu-nicated.

Bureaucratic inhibitions are often reflected in discrepancies among noramlly functioning but contradictory processes. Rosner, for example, studied the apparent contradiction between administra-tive controls and organizational innovation in 24 short-term, volun-tary nonteaching hospitals. She found support for two hypotheses: (1) that innovation varies inversely with activities control because activities control reduces the search for new programs and abridges the individual's capacity and incentive to innovate; and (2) that inno-vation varies directly with the visibility of consequences, since such visibility permits the evaluation of the innovation's effect on goal achievement, and allows the organization to reward and en-courage successful innovators.[5]

THE ROLE OF TECHNOLOGICAL CHANGE

In bureaucracies such as Victory Hospital, technological change finds greater support, readier adoption, and smoother im-plementation than does organizational or managerial change not directly rooted in technology. Victory was found to be strongest in technological, task oriented, or proocdural change, and weakest in managerial or people-oriented change. Experience in the former area does not automatically imply skills in the latter, even though the general processes depicted in our basic model of change and innovation are basically the same for both. This is not surprising, but it should be a matter of further research for it is in the area of organization and management behavior that Victory found its ability to innovate most limited. For example, there were in use no truly advanced management methods, such as programs for organization development or management by objectives.

The observations at Victory yield several reasons for this. One is that technological change is more readily justified. The hospital needs to keep up with other hospitals and with the demands of physicians and patients. Economic or cost-benefit factors predominate in the decision making. As long as economic factors permit, technological changes will occur, often without undue concern for their human relations consequences. But managerial or organizational changes are harder to justify, for strategies, cost, and results are harder to measure. Furthermore, the protests, resistances, and hesitancies due to human attitudes and emotions are more easily overcome by the logics and economics of technology, whereas other types of change are more likely to founder on the shoals of uncertainty and self-interest. It is easier to install a new brain scanner than a system of management by objectives.

Another reason why technological change is easier is that it is buffered within the technological core by interdependencies within and among the technological groups. Although these interdependencies may sometimes be dysfunctional with regard to change, they can also be a source of mutual support in areas of technological improvement.

Yet the progress of technological change is not always smooth, nor are the economic justifications always correct. To begin with, the concept of technology is not as definite or unambiguous as the term implies. Technology is best defined broadly as including all the characteristics of the organization's inputs, transformation activities, and the outputs.[6] Furthermore, the different dimensions of technology vary, depending on the observer's perspective. Physicians' views differ from those of administrators, for example.[7] Although technology is one of the prime determinants of task and organizational structure, there is ample room for disagreement over the proper ways to perform and distribute the hospital's work. Therefore, conflict and tensions arise between physicians, administrators, technologists, and other groups in the allied health professions.

One example will suffice to illustrate how the use of cost justifications alone for technological change can go astray. In 1972, Congress enacted a social security bill containing a supposedly inexpensive provision to pay the medical costs of kidney dialysis and transplants for several thousand patients. The assumption was that lower-cost home treatments would in many cases replace hospital care. But with federal funding, hospitalization increased. A program expected to cost $250 million a year mushroomed to over $1 billion in 1977, and this figure is expected to double by 1982. Such results can have enormous impacts on the hospital, but they also lead to questions about the advancing technology of medicine, doubts about the financing and encouragement of innovation by the government, and the eventual possibility of control over the pace and extent of innovation through the development of "standards." However, since it is unlikely that the tide of medical innovation can be stopped, the trend for better evaluation and planning and the control of proliferation for reasons of status or profit may be welcomed. The hospital's role in technological change will be very much under review in the future, and hospital administrators and their medical-technical staffs will be caught up in the tensions thereby produced. [8]

Drucker, focusing on dialysis problems as an example, gives us an additional insight, namely, that costly technology often is not healing; rather, it is a way of postponing death. Hence the decision makers are not only faced with questions of economics and cost, for their decisions are ultimately problems of ethics. Economics is a restraint. The decision is spiritual, not medical. [9]

It is important to stress one additional dimension of the problem of technological change, namely, that there are psychoanalytical overtones in innovative or noninnovative performance. The bureaucratic impulses in hospital management and organization, to the extent that they are heeded, speak for order, control, routinization, and systematic procedures. In the hospital setting, it is therefore possible that the spokesmen for and progenitors of technology will dominate the system. The system they prefer will be bureaucratic. According to Zaleznik and Kets de Vries, there is a necessary mix of technocrats who design the system of compliers, who do the work they are told to do:

> Compulsive subordinacy and passivity in character
> structure contain features that support a technologi-
> cally oriented society. In such a society, the inno-
> vations come from a select portion of the populations,
> usually well-educated people trained in the sciences
> and engineering. The technocrats design the system,
> which will work only if the people who man the ma-
> chines and the assembly lines are willing to comply with
> the programs. If people try to innovate, to express
> their individuality, or to "malinger," they reduce rather
> than improve the effectiveness of technological systems.
> Consequently, their willingness to comply is more im-
> portant than their active motivation to create, achieve,
> or express themselves. The complying person is often
> the compulsive individual, for whom repetitive work
> may be a release from anxiety and doubt of thought,
> fantasy, and action. [10]

Our next task is to examine some directions by which hospital administrators and other health care professionals may overcome bureaucratic limitations and advance beyond the limitations of technological change. The central approach is called a proactive strategy of administration.

TOWARD A PROACTIVE APPROACH TO HOSPITAL ADMINISTRATION

Hospitals should, on the face of things, be innovative. They face not only external pressures for innovation from public demands for more, better, and cheaper services, and the forces generated by other parts of the health care system, but also a host of internal pressures from well-educated, highly trained employees who value autonomy in their work and are spurred by patient care motives. But bureaucracy's strong foothold of centralized policies and rigid management structures can be changed.

An alternative to bureaucracy and its constraints is to develop a more open system which encourages use of participative management. This requires alterations in management styles and in the attitudinal and value systems of people. Since the necessary incentives for doing so are limited, the hospital has to overcome great odds to accomplish this kind of change. Yet, the members of the hospital's organization are its source of strength as well as of problems. The lack of incentives for innovation can be met by more creative managerial action designed to free the bureaucracy of constraints on ideation, adoption, and implementation of change.

Without discarding bureaucracy blindly and completely, the hospital can undertake a planned evolution in management style that rejects self-protective, dehumanizing leadership and minimizes the use of mechanisms designed to assure certainty of control, predictability of behavior, orderly procedure, and conformity of individuals to the status quo. Open systems are receptive to ideas, to change, to human needs and interests, and to the external environment. The open-system view seems natural when aligned against the fact that a hospital is after all a federation of interest groups with appropriate claims to autonomy. The open system respects the individual; the hierarchy is not worshiped; nor are rigid, sacrosanct domains formed around vested interests. The element of trust developed around common interests in missions and in problem solving replaces the fears and lack of courage that attend adherence to bureaucratic concepts.[11]

A case for an open-system approach to hospital management can be supported by recognizing the propensity of bureaucratic stability and control over time to become burdensome and inappropriate. Stability stifles innovation and discourages creativity for only a time; the needs of people for fun, excitement, and achievement sooner or later come to override the forces of stability, with mounting pressures for change. Demands from external sources become too heavy to ignore. But since there are also limits to change that will eventually come into play, we see a circular, interactive process of alternating change, assessment, and stability.

It has been alleged that innovation and change cannot be controlled or managed.[12] This thesis is contradicted by the behavior observed in this study, for we have seen that the principal actors in a hospital organization recognize the need for innovation and change, and indeed attempt to influence these processes. Yet for all the innovation and change at Victory, it remains an institution much like others of its general class. It is modern, successful, and well respected. On most standards of evaluation, it would rank high compared to similar institutions. However, it has found no breakthrough innovations that give it thrust and momentum beyond the maintenance of organizational solvency and professional competence.

Perhaps this is enough to ask of a hospital. However, when this finding is viewed in the light of momentous and intense pressures of rising costs, increased service demands, and the presence of the hospital as a new center of gravity in the health care system as a whole, we may well question whether sufficient progress is possible without a deliberately managed focus on innovation and creativity.

Some will argue that change and innovation follow a measured pace of their own, constituting an inevitability beyond management's tampering. Kaufman, for example, argues that in most organizations, change is gradual, and that the number, magnitude, and importance of changes are kept within rather narrow limits over any comparatively short period, such as a generation. Thus, change occurs by the accretion of small modifications of existing, ongoing systems. This to him is the way the world is ordered.[13] This also was the way Victory's organization was ordered. In so ordering itself, Victory Hospital was able to satisfy most of the immediate demands upon it. But it fell short of maximizing its larger potential for innovation and change.

Zaleznik and Kets de Vries describe how organizations move historically through three basic leadership strategies: homeostatic, mediative, and proactive. A homeostatic strategy addresses the need for preserving the organization to insure internal stability and continuity in the face of internal forces of disruption. A mediative strategy aims at changes in the organization arising out of the impact of external pressures. A proactive strategy moves the organization aggressively to induce changes in the environment through the creative use of its resources. Accordingly, proactivity is the strategy of major innovation and change. Victory's strategy was primarily mediative, a level sufficient to earn it a solid reputation for respectable and able management. It is only when we compare this strategy to the enormous tasks at hand that we can judge the need for a proactive strategy.[14]

One difficulty with the proactive strategy is that it tends to induce resistance, aggression, and sometimes outright hostility within the organization. It forces the extensive disruption of internal relations among members of the organization by shifting its aims from internal problems to the taking of aggressive initiatives against the environment. Ambiguities arise, risks increase, uncertainties abound. Major domains of entrenched interests are assaulted, and it becomes more difficult to defend the status quo on the grounds that an adequate effort has been made to meet reasonable demands. Consequently, the need for resourcefulness, stamina, and effective interpersonal relations skills on the part of administrators is greatly increased. The managers in Victory Hospital were not practiced in coping with tensions, stress, resistance, or aggression arising out of change. They were easily deflected from innovative efforts by the strike threats, and the extensive evaluation mechanisms served to assure that proposed changes would not be seriously disruptive—that they would "fit in" with current operations. Resistance was not directly confronted so as to support innovative efforts; instead, it was used along with permissiveness, voting, and experimentation to prolong the diffusion and implementation processes. Replacements for departing managers were deliberately designed to foster a return to equanimity and conservative views. These limits to courageous innovation in the guise of permissiveness or allowances for professional autonomies served to limit innovations and changes to those most readily accepted by vested interests.

The tasks and responsibilities of a mediative strategy are in themselves so demanding on managers that it is not surprising to find little impetus for a proactive strategy. To embark upon such a strategy requires the hospital to shed the trappings of tradition, to redefine its problems in very long-range terms, and to unshackle its managers from at least some of the bureaucratic constraints that limit or delay innovative efforts to change.

How does the hospital administrator move from a mediative to a proactive strategy? Placed in position by the bureaucracy, the administrator deals with protected turfs—domains of the powerful who are supported by professional and technical interest groups.

Those same groups, too, may aid the would-be change agent on the hospital's staff. Therefore the administrator, in a leadership role, must confront both the demands for stability and the demands for change. The administration's role is thus a pivotal one in the interplay of political forces within and without the organization.

Politics is essentially a game in which the astute use of power counts most.[15] Not everything that goes on in an organization can be managed. Managers are selective in what they try to manage. Some innovation and change may be desirable and necessary; some is undesirable and unnecessary. Since decisions have to be made, and since one cannot ignore organizational politics in decision making, one must view innovation and change at least in part in the light of their relation to organizational politics.

Granting the administrator's appreciation of the need for political adroitness, this study makes it possible to suggest three main strategies designed to move the hospital organization from a mediative strategy to a more proactive one:

1. Identify and reward creative people, and include the capacity for change and innovation as a criterion for selection and placement.

2. Develop an organization system that gives creative people, designated change agents, and boundary spanners adequate opportunities and challenges.

3. Consider a total strategy such as an organization development program or a management by objectives program designed to utilize the best of what is known by behavioral scientists.

This threefold strategy was not apparent in Victory Hospital. Innovation and change in Victory were left mainly to the random efforts of individuals with other primary preoccupations. No one was charged solely with planning for innovation and change, and only two of the five top administrators professed solid orientation for change. There were no staff groups to assist would-be change agents or to generate change. There is little doubt that hospitals can benefit from a more explicit recognition of the need to manage change and innovation. This recognition would be reflected in specific administrative responsibilities allocated to this function, so that the question of who gives time and attention to them would be more apparent.

Even in the absence of staff units for planning and developing change and the like, the hospital organization can identify its innovative, creative persons for the purpose of freeing them for their best efforts. Guetzkow has indicated that identifying idea persons allows them to be placed strategically in the organization where they can benefit from organization slack and communicate better with those in the organization who can gain from their creativity. In fact, identifying the innovator tends to increase his potential for creativity because such roles set up reciprocal expectations among members of the organization. Since creative individuals may tend to isolate themselves, or to be cold-shouldered by bureaucrats, it is imperative to put them where they are accessible and available so the whole organization can tap this resource.[16]

The matter of hiring specific persons for the purpose of bringing about change is controversial. In industry, and in some hospitals, troubleshooters are brought in to wield a heavy ax, and to shake things up in a turnaround situation. Many hospitals are not waiting for crises of finance or other problems to bring in bright and able people with MBAs, MHAs, or MPHs and giving them assignments as change agents. This strategy is uncomfortable to vested interests, and it will not work where higher administration itself is the root cause of mismanagement. The overall quality of management has its impact on change. If the hospital becomes financially bankrupt, among the multitude of causes could be administrative drift—where managers cease to manage and simply react to internal or external stimuli.[17]

Thus, the first strategy, that of identifying existing and potential change agents and innovators, implies the conferring of the power of discretionary change. Discretionary change, if recognized as such, engenders resistance from those who value the status quo. Therefore the administrator's strategy wherever possible is to convert discretionary change into the image of inevitable change, to gain acquiescence. He can also use legitimate power to force compliance with change, but the best kind of "inevitable" change is that which can be attributed to outsiders or outside forces. Therefore effective boundary spanners are essential, and the more open the system, the more likely it is that boundary spanners will be active in the change process.[18] As the "wave of the future" washes over an organization, the outcomes depend on the skills, insights, and leadership abilities of the administrator and other change agents.

Crozier has argued that the freedom and discretion of the innovative figure require the strict ritualism of those at lower levels and the submissiveness of those at middle levels. Those at the lower levels are required to support the bureaucracy by enforcing rules without leeway, but the dysfunctions this creates point to the need for innovators. Middle managers act as transmission links, but the innovator has the discretion to make adjustments, thereby acquiring power and prestige. Intermediate officials are "too involved in the discussion of arbitrary exceptions to rules and in the resetting of the rules to adopt the ritualist and rebellious attitudes

of their subordinates, but too helpless themselves to assume responsibilities." Further, the power of discretion is so exceptional
that it must be removed from face-to-face relationships and sur-
rounded by an aura of awe and submissiveness.[19]

What Crozier's views imply for the hospital administrator is
that he must come to terms in his management style and philosophy
with the hierarchical aspects of the hospital organization. The roles
of the bureaucrat, the self-satisfied person, the honored innovator,
the submissive assistant, and the ritualistic minion come together
in any managerial focus on innovation and change. If bureaucratic
elements are stable and power lies in role enforcement, higher
levels of innovation and change may be precluded. In the enlarge-
ment of the pool of innovators and change agents with discretionary
powers are great possibilities for innovation and change.

The second strategy involves developing organization structures that assign discretionary powers to formally designated change
agents. These should include staff units capable of giving high
visibility to change agents, providing experts with an organizational
base, and establishing legitimate, challenging opportunities, and
commensurate rewards. Staff units also provide status and resources for creative people. These units should be located at the
top echelon of the hospital. They consist of planners, idea people,
persuaders, and pools of expertise on which other units can draw.
Such groups need not be large to be effective; they do increase an
organization's overhead costs. But to achieve greater innovation
and change, the costs may be viewed as investments in long-range
planning.

It should be noted that staff units, such as those for planning,
organizational development, or personnel and labor relations, perform functions and services other than those of innovation and
change. The administrator should manage staff groups in such a
way as to enhance the activities that lead to improved innovation
and change.

The third strategy is an extension of the logic of the first two
strategies. A total organization approach is required for moving
most effectively from the breaucratic to an open system view, and
from mediative to proactive management. Total approaches come
in many forms, but the most common examples are programs for
management by objectives (MBO) and for organization development
(OD). Neither program is a panacea, but each is a way of applying
behavioral science knowledge to the development of open-system
management styles, which in turn lead to better opportunities for
managing innovation and change.

In Victory, the top administrators espoused an MBO approach.
On examination, however, this was more a verbal posture than an

actual program. A fully operative MBO plan involves the mutual development of objectives, joint planning by supervisors and subordinates, and performance evaluations based on achievement of planned goals.[20] Instead, Victory's managers saw MBO more as a reporting and record system than as a sharing of goal planning. It was not a complete program, and it did not entail systematic performance-based appraisals.

The organization development approach (OD) is even rarer in hospitals than MBO programs. Wiesbord argues that such programs have not proved feasible in hospitals.[21] His arguments are unconvincing, since there is so little evidence of serious trials. Also, properly managed organization development programs are tailormade for specific settings. Therefore it is likely that, in the overall concept of OD, there are potentials of enormous benefit for hospitals if there exists a serious intent to modify the bureaucracy to achieve better innovation and change.

OD is a program which recognizes that to bring about lasting changes in individual attitudes and performance, work must also be done both on organization structure and the attitudinal climate. This kind of total approach stresses involvement and participation in planning, making changes, and evaluating results. These programs entail long-run commitments, legitimation by the top leadership, and patience in dealing with inevitable setbacks and difficulties. Generally, a behavioral science consultant is needed to help steer the course of the several evolutionary stages, to provide knowledge and techniques, and to buffer the resistances that occur.[22]

In sum, an OD program would in itself constitute an innovation for the hospital. It also would lay the groundwork for the nurture of innovation and change in all aspects of the organization. By undertaking an OD program, the hospital would undergo a learning process that is essential to the maintenance of its capacity to innovate and change. In this process, the administrator can build up the expectations of change by inculcating in the organizational climate such beliefs as "we are a change-oriented place," or "we are growing." As long as the ends toward which change is directed are worthy and rational, progress will be made.

One sign that modifications to bureaucratic structures and management styles are progressing into the hospital arena is found in the wider attention now being paid to matrix organization. Matrix organization is a structural design that requires the development of open-system thinking, and for maximum effectiveness also requires the use of advanced behavioral science knowledge and techniques. Matrix designs are highly applicable in high technology organizations, such as hospitals.[23]

Matrix structure is defined as an organization that employs a multiple command structure and related support mechanisms, together with related management procedures and styles.[24] It is often combined with bureaucratic structures and with project management. While a hierarchy is still present, matrix organization consists of a lateral structure of support service units, and a vertical structure of project or operating units.

Matrix organization combined with project or task force units involves the use of project or unit directors, and teams consisting of selected specialists whose capabilities are needed in the project. The project is long-term, but personnel assignments to it are temporary. When the project is finished, all personnel are reassigned. When a more permanent matrix structure is utilized, such as in nursing services, the problems of reassignment do not occur, but the organization benefits by identifying the main operating units and the service units that contribute to their work. Since matrix structures tend to decentralize authority and responsibility and to put service units on a consultative basis, it opens the organization up and provides greater flexibility and propensity for change than is possible in traditional bureaucracies.

Figure 12.1 provides a schematic illustration of a matrix structure that could be designed for hospitals. It shows the multiple-command system, with operating units on the vertical dimension and the supporting units on the horizontal dimension. The duplication of functions entailed in this structure raises cost considerations that would have to be offset by gains in flexibility, adaptability, and mobility of human resources.

In many ways, Victory and other hospitals operate like a matrix organization despite their ostensible bureaucratic tendencies. Moving to a more proactive management and a matrix or other open-system structure would bring the heretofore submerged objectives of change and innovation out into the open.

An overall assessment of the findings of this exploratory study indicates that in effect two different structural patterns of organization are required for the effective management of innovation and change. Duncan has postulated the utility of two-tier, dual patterns of organization for purposes of innovation, so that each part of the design can be focused on phases of innovation it is best able to perform.[25] For the creation of change opportunities, for problem-solving capability, for drawing out and nurturing ideas, and for creative responses to outside needs and pressures, the open-system, flexible organization design is best. For adopting, testing, evaluating, and establishing the resulting changes and ideas, bureaucratic processes are best.

FIGURE 12.1

Illustrative Matrix Structure

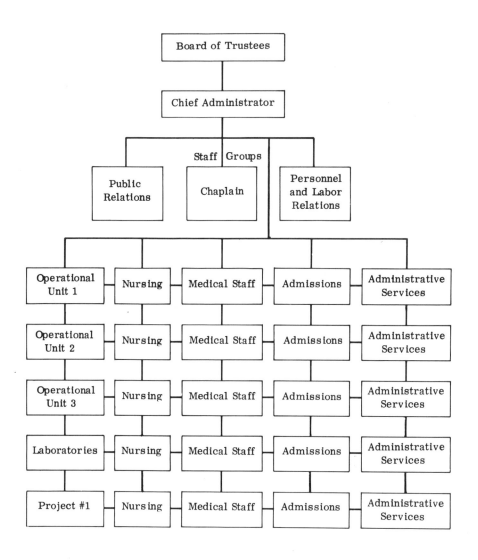

Source: Constructed by the author.

The dual pattern has the advantage of more clearly recognizing the existence of resources within the lower echelons of an organization, and making it possible to bring forth the creative ideas of "marginal" members of the organization. However, it is still an unresolved question whether persons in marginal roles in society or in organizations more readily devise or adopt innovations than those higher in status or position. Marginal persons are variously described as "submerged," "peripheral," "alienated," "powerless," or "socially disaffected." Presumably, they would innovate from desperation and undertake high risk with relatively little to lose from failure. In 1960, however, Menzel observed that the classical notion that innovations are most readily adopted by marginal people appeared to be contradicted by findings in studies of the adoption of new drugs by physicians. This led him to suggest that innovations of different kinds find readiest adoption in different positions of the social structure, and that there are complex intervening variables between social position and the acceptance of an innovation. [26]

Borman, however, studied two dimensions of marginality—the notion of marginal segments in society coupled with the marginal aspects of culture, finding marginality a productive locus of innovation. The marginal aspects of culture are those which are considered frivolous or nonutilitarian, such as play, recreation, or the creative activities in art, science, and philosophy. Borman studied an innovation in a large mental hospital in which a patient council was established by socially marginal professionals working in the "culturally frivolous" activities of play and anthropological research. The innovation was directed toward backward, chronically ill patients who were clearly marginal. Over a six-year period, however, the effects of the innovation spread to less marginal professionals and less marginal patients, meeting with increasing success. The implications for organizational change of the two roles studied (anthropology researchers and recreation specialists) were described by Borman as follows:

> The roles . . . can be considered underdefined. Such roles, in Gunder Frank's terms, permit individuals actively to take the determination of their own and others' destines into their own hands, [resulting] in many different ad hoc responses to situations in which guiding norms either do not exist or are not enforceable by existing sanctions. These roles contrast with the prevailing "well-defined" roles of most bureaucratic organizations which prohibit individual initiative and make ritual role performance easy, if not mandatory. [27]

The research at Victory found no strong negative evidence as to the ability of marginal persons in administrative roles to contribute to innovation and change. There were differences as to level in the organization and as to functional responsibilities. It may be suggested, however, that marginality may be of less significance in hospitals because of the way all roles, marginal or otherwise, incorporate a strong ethos of patient care. The dual structure, however, may well serve to encourage creativity among marginal persons.

Creativity is an attribute of good leadership. Victory's chaplain, for example, saw creativity of different kinds at different levels, and the temptation of many to give lip service to the idea of creativity without being able or willing to actualize their creative urges:

> Chaplain: . . . a lot of people just talk about creativity.
> You have people that talk ideas all the time. But I
> think they only give lip service to it. They play the
> role of presenting good ideas, but they can't actualize
> any ideas. A good leader has to hustle to keep up and
> project new ideas into the organization. That's better
> than just pulling the idea along with him.
> Interviewer: Maybe the same person can't play all the
> roles necessary to creativity and innovation.
> Chaplain: Yes, that's right. I think the idea generator
> often cannot go beyond that. Then you have others
> who are capable of operationalizing the idea, and
> still a third set of people who give it the ultimate
> testing and acceptance, and put the idea to work. A
> good analogy is in the field of architecture where you
> have the architect, the contractor, and the building
> supply people. Each one has a limit to his creativity
> that is prescribed by the work he is doing and the nature of the field he is in. You can't expect a building
> supply person to supply a creative idea about the
> architecture. What is important is developing the
> relationships between the elements, such as between
> physicians and others in the health care field.
> Interviewer: What would you think the fate of a pretty
> good idea would be in this organization generally?
> Chaplain: That depends on where it originates and who
> the people are who are going to pick it up and run
> with the ball. Some people in this organization have
> a role and status and a reputation such that an idea
> of theirs will carry more weight than ideas from

anyone else. I'm sure that if a black maintenance
or kitchen employee came up with a good idea, it
wouldn't have nearly the same reception and would
take a lot longer to come into existence if he is putting it out than if it comes from somebody higher up.
In order to get an idea across, one has to get powerful allies to help push the idea up.

T. S. Eliot has reinforced the chaplain's views in the following statement:

A vision however arrived at, demands realization in
some concrete form. At every level of management we
need a rediscovery of the value of the individual imagination and rekindling of that passion for humane purposes
which is the authentic light of leadership. To manage is
to lead, and to lead others requires that one enlist the
emotions of others to share a vision as their own. If
that is not an art, then nothing is.[28]

CONCLUSION

Gertrude Stein has remarked that anything truly original must
have a touch of ugliness because it has not had a chance to be honed
to the elegance that comes with refinement.[29] This epitomizes the
processes of innovation and change as observed in Victory and
other hospitals. New and original ideas are continuously being
refined so that their ugliness is transformed. Our theoretical
understanding of this process is still all too limited.

What we have now are only partial theories and segments or
pieces of research. The vast jungle of general organization theory
to which hospital organization theory is allied is unstable and in a
state of transition. Yet a general theory of organization will ultimately be needed to form the base for hospital organization theory.
In turn, the theory of innovation and change in hospitals depends
heavily on both general theory and the theory of hospital organization.
Theoretical conceptualization and empirical research are advancing
in all these areas, but formidable problems of integration remain.
Convergencies are appearing that should encourage researchers
and practitioners alike to join each other in pursuing an integration
of theories and practices.

NOTES

1. James Q. Wilson, "Innovation in Organization: Notes Toward a Theory," in Approaches to Organizational Design, ed. James D. Thompson (Pittsburgh: University of Pittsburgh Press, 1966), pp. 195-218.

2. Ibid.

3. Herbert Kaufman, The Limits of Organizational Change (University: University of Alabama Press, 1971).

4. Victor A. Thompson, "How Scientific Management Thwarts Innovation," Trans-Action, June 1968, pp. 51-55.

5. Marian M. Rosner, "Administrative Controls and Innovation," Behavioral Sciences 13, no. 1 (January 1968): 36-43.

6. W. Richard Scott, "Professionals in Hospitals: Technology and the Organization of Work," in Organization Research on Health Institutions, ed. Basil S. Georgopoulis (Ann Arbor: Institute for Social Research, University of Michigan, 1972), pp. 145-46.

7. Ibid., p. 156.

8. Jonathan Spivak, "Medical Planners Seek to Balance Costs and Benefits," Wall Street Journal, November 14, 1977, p. 8.

9. Interview with Peter F. Drucker, Federation of American Hospitals Review, February 1978, p. 39.

10. Abraham Zaleznik and Manfred F. R. Kets de Vries, Power and the Corporate Mind (Boston: Houghton Mifflin, 1975), p. 159.

11. Readers who wish to augment their understanding of open systems are encouraged to consult the following basic works: Daniel Katz and Robert Kahn, The Social Psychology of Organizations, 2nd ed. (New York: Wiley, 1978); John G. Maurer, ed., Readings in Organizational Theory: Open System Approaches (New York: Random House, 1971); Tom Burns and G. M. Stalker, The Management of Innovation (Chicago: Quadrangle Books, 1962).

12. Samuel Globe, Gerard W. Levy, and Charles M. Schwartz, "Key Factors and Events in the Innovation Process," International Journal of Research Management 16, no. 4 (July 1973): 8-15.

13. Kaufman, op. cit.

14. Zaleznik and Kets de Vries, op. cit., p. 31.

15. Anthony T. Cobb, "The Politics of Innovation," Annual Proceedings, Southeast Division, American Institute of Decision Sciences 8th Annual Meeting, 1978.

16. Harold Guetzkow, "The Creative Person in Organizations," in The Creative Organization, ed. Gary A. Steiner (Chicago: University of Chicago Press, 1965), pp. 43-44.

17. Gary E. Stone, "Can Hospitals Be Managed?" MBA, March 1976.

18. See, for example, Michael L. Tushman, "Special Boundary Roles in the Innovation Process," Administrative Science Quarterly 22 (December 1977): 587-605.

19. Michel Crozier, The Bureaucratic Phenomenon (Chicago: University of Chicago Press, 1964), p. 202.

20. For a full description of MBO, see George S. Odiorne, Management by Objectives (New York: Pitman, 1965); and Stephen J. Carroll and Henry L. Tosi, Management by Objectives: Applications and Research (New York: Macmillan, 1973). See also Fred Luthans and Jerry Sellentin, "MBO in Hospitals: A Step Toward Accountability," The Personnel Administrator 21 (October 1976): 42-45; and Herbert R. Hand and A. Thomas Hollingsworth, "Tailoring MBO to Hospitals," Business Horizons, February 1975, pp. 45-52.

21. Marvin R. Wiesbord, "Why Organization Development Hasn't Worked (So Far) in Medical Centers," Health Care Management Review, Spring 1976, pp. 17-28.

22. For further information, see Paul R. Lawrence and Jay W. Lorsch, Developing Organizations: Diagnosis and Action (Reading, Mass.: Addison-Wesley, 1969); Richard Beckhard, Organization Development: Strategies and Models (Reading, Mass.: Addison-Wesley, 1969); Wendell L. French and Cecil H. Bell, Jr., Organization Development: Behavioral Science Interventions for Organizational Improvement (Englewood Cliffs, N.J.: Prentice-Hall, 1973).

23. Terence F. Moore and B. E. Lorimer, "The Matrix Organization on Business and Health Care Institutions: A Comparison," Hospital and Health Services Administration 21 (Fall 1976): 26-34; Duncan Neuhauser, "The Hospital as a Matrix Organization," Hospital Administration 17 (Fall 1972): 8-25; G. Vaugn Johnson and Sherman Tingey, "Matrix Organization: Blueprint of Nursing Care Organization," Hospital and Health Services Administration 21 (Winter 1976): 27-39.

24. Stanley M. Davis and Paul R. Lawrence, Matrix (Reading, Mass.: Addison-Wesley, 1977).

25. Robert J. Duncan, "The Ambidextrous Organization: Designing Dual Structures for Innovation," in The Management of Organization Design: Strategies and Implementations, ed. Ralph H. Kilmann, Louis R. Pondy, and Dennis L. Slevin, vol. I (New York: Elsevier North-Holland, 1976).

26. Herbert Menzel, "Innovation, Integration, and Marginality: A Survey of Physicians," American Sociological Review 25 (1960): 704-13.

27. Leonard D. Borman, "The Marginal Route of a Mental Hospital Innovation," Human Organization 29 (1970): 63-69. See

also A. Gunder Frank, "Administrative Role Definition and Social Change," Human Organization 22 (Winter 1963-64): 238-42.

28. T. S. Eliot, quoted in Henry M. Boettinger, "Is Management Really an Art?" Harvard Business Review, January-February 1975, pp. 63-64.

29. Quoted by Charles Eames in Owen Gingrich, "A Conversation with Charles Eames, " American Scholar 46 (Summer 1977): 329.

NOTES ON RESEARCH METHODOLOGY

Victory Hospital was an attractive research site, for it exhibited interesting patterns of innovation and change. It was large enough to have significant management activities and problems; it attracted a wide range of experienced managerial, technical, and medical talent. And, most important of all, its managers and administrators were exceptionally cooperative and tolerant of the interventions of the researchers. The receptivity of hospitals to the research investigations of behavioral scientists is a relatively recent development. It is fortunate that hospitals such as Victory are increasingly open to the inquiries of sociologists, psychologists, applied anthropologists, economists, and social psychologists. Like Victory, they are becoming accustomed to research interventions, to probing analyses, and to the scholarly publication of the findings. This appears to be true even where practical payoffs are minimal and in any case cannot be guaranteed by the researcher.

The primary data utilized in this study consisted of the contents of a total of 72 depth interviews. Fifty-four of these were with managers from Victory Hospital. Eight preliminary interviews and 10 additional interviews were obtained from the chief administrators in nearby hospitals. Secondary data were also obtained from published research reports, from press clippings about Norfield and Victory, and from documents and papers provided by Norfield and Victory. Originally conceived as an intensive case study of a single hospital, additional funding made it possible to broaden the study at several points following the first two years of field work.

These methods of research posed the problem of analyzing an enormous quantity of qualitative data generated by the interviews. This task involved two interrelated procedures: (1) determining the substantive issues to serve as a structure for the coding process and (2) establishing a uniform coding procedure providing ready access to the information assigned to the selected categories of data. The first step was to develop the substantive categories of analysis. Following methods suggested by Glaser and Strauss,[1] eight main categories and their relevant dimensions were established. The content of the categories, in the form of dimensions, was developed from continuing examinations of the accumulating interview data and a study of the literature of organizational innovation and change.

The following identifying names were given to the eight categories: organizational framework, ideation, capabilities of people, change processes, evaluation and assessment process, adoption process, diffusion-implementation process, and role behaviors.

Each category was described by a brief conceptual statement, and a number of analytical properties were hypothesized for each category. The interviews were then examined for coherent passages, called "bits." A bit consists of related portions of dialog between interviewer and subject, or a paragraph of observations. The contents of a bit were allocated on the basis of their fit to issues or problems rather than to discrete events. The final step was to code each bit into one or more appropriate categories and to code for each bit the dimensions within the category. A complete listing of the categories and dimensions is included in Appendix D.

During the analysis, a large number of bits were reassigned to more appropriate categories. Some of the hypothesized dimensions within categories did not include sufficient or useful data. These were discarded or consolidated with other dimensions. Nevertheless, the coding system successfully fulfilled its twin functions of access and systematic ordering of data.

One problem of analyzing the data and reporting the findings was caused by the way that a given event or issue frequently pervaded several interviews over the two-year period, involving different persons with varying degrees of involvement and knowledge. It would have been possible to analyze the data by bringing together all the material on each specific major event or activity. Instead, it was decided to base the analysis on managerial or organizational issues and theory. This resulted in dividing major events into bits designed to explicate and illustrate particular theoretical or practical problems. Thus, for example, the events, activities, and attitudes of people in the process of acquiring a new brain wave scanner are not analyzed in one place, but rather in several places throughout the book.

The open-ended, unstructured nature of the field methods followed in the study of Victory Hospital were unfamiliar to the informants. Nevertheless, they responded clearly and confidently to the interviewers' queries. They were told that the study was exploratory and that the researcher's aim was to connect parts of the real world of hospital management to emergent concepts in the research literature on managerial innovation and change. No evidence of hostility, antagonism, or abnormal resistance was encountered. On the contrary, rapport between the interviewers and the informants was high, and it continued to be so throughout the study. There were no restrictions placed on the observations, questions, or the inspection of documents, records, and working papers.

From the beginning, it was decided to take a holistic view of the hospital rather than to select certain parts for special emphasis.

The modern hospital represents a complex affiliation of a wide spectrum of occupations and professions, each deserving careful study in its own right. However, to study all the processes through which these groups in a hospital are linked would have been a lengthy and costly task. Therefore, a narrowing but integrative conceptual focus on managerial innovation and change was selected as a way of studying the hospital as a unit, while at the same time giving the study a depth of penetration. This approach permitted the observation of the interacting roles, professions, occupations, and tasks of members and clients of the organization, as well as of the connective tissues among them.

The methods used in this study, principally interviewing and observation, were chiefly those of sociology and applied anthropology. They were chiefly clinical in character. The explorations began with concepts, ideas, basic generalizations, and hypotheses prevalent in or deducible from available writings. An interviewing protocol, included as Appendix C, was devised to systematize the interviewing procedures and to pose the exploratory questions for the initial interviews. These protocols were useful in training and coordinating the work of the two interviewers who assisted the author in the data collection phases of the study.

Depth interviewing techniques utilizing open-ended questions led to the collection of a large amount of anecdotal, descriptive material. Nearly all of the administrators at the top two levels at Victory were interviewed at least twice, and the chief administrator was interviewed six times. Although the first interviews were patterned similarly, in accordance with the protocols, the repeat interviews varied more widely to permit going into greater depth on specific issues or problems in the particular informant's domain of interest or responsibility. Thus, the interviewers followed a flexible approach that permitted the pursuit of lines of inquiry not fully anticipated in the early planning.

Recorders were not used during actual interviews, but the researchers, with the permission of informants, took ample notes. Following each interview, the material was recorded as fully as possible, in dialog form, in the order the information emerged during the interview. An effort was made to record the dialog of both interviewer and interviewee as close to verbatim as possible, but clearly this idea can only be approximated. The resulting effect was to obtain real-life accounts of attitudes, events, and perspectives phrased in the lively but often repetitious and ungrammatical language of ordinary discourse. The coding and subsequent analysis of data for presentation in this book were accomplished in accordance with widely used field work and qualitative analysis techniques derived from the sources listed at the end of this appendix.

It is recognized that a case study of this type has limitations, an important one being the lack of a base for generalizing propositions and predictions to other hospitals, even those of a type similar to Victory. Yet hospital and other health care practitioners can see for themselves the dynamic processes of innovation and change in a hospital typical of many. Researchers may derive useful hypotheses and general propositions for cross-sectional comparative research that can be tested in further studies. The case study approach was selected to allow for depth and breadth of penetration, for meticulous and complete description of relevant forces at work, and for providing a richer base from which to evolve hypotheses and propositions.

With respect to research on innovation, Becker and Whisler have pointed out that the cross-sectional studies of a number of organizations or organizational units, with attempts to establish statistical relationships between selected inputs and outputs, have been quite disappointing. Such methods assume innovation to be a single intervening variable, whereas innovation appears more likely to be a complex process involving a number of critical variables. This leads to the need for longitudinal analysis and for intensive case studies.[2] This study of Victory reported here represents an effort in this direction.

Clinical investigation was chosen in preference to survey research chiefly because of its notable absence in the repertory of hospital management research, and because of the need for the immersion of field researchers into the intimacies of hospital organization life. The clinical approach, with its emphasis on interviewing and observation, seeks to identify and explain nuances in the hospital culture that lie beyond the reach of traditional survey research or cross-sectional comparisons. One thus confronts, as a researcher, the import of his personal relationships to the subjects of his studies. This has been eloquently stated by Mauksch:

> With his desire to chart the unique characteristics of
> his objects of study, and to observe and understand
> the unique features of the norms, customs, and be-
> havior of the investigated environment, he must also
> establish his own relationships to this world, come
> to terms with his own feelings and values, and do so
> in consideration of the success of his enterprise.[3]

An important question is whether hospitals can be treated like any other organization for the purpose of theory and its applications. Heydebrand calls the hospital "the prototype of modern work organization."[4] Certainly, the service sector of an economy, of which the hospital is part, is the largest and fastest growing sector. Yet many believe that the hospital should be studied in its own right as a unique type of institution. Comparative theory and research can then be brought to bear to discover the similarities and differences between hospitals and other types of organizations. Critics allege that present-day research in hospitals is naive, simplistic, and repetitious without being replicative. No doubt much of it is. We do need to stop being naive and reinventing the managerial wheel. Yet there remains a great need for studies of the microcosm of the hospital—its people, their values, and their interests. Merely borrowing concepts and methods from other disciplines, though helpful, is not enough. Breakthroughs are more likely if we grapple directly with the hospital and its problems.

The methods used in this study were primarily derived from the exceptionally valuable treatise by Glaser and Strauss.[5] They advance a qualitative methodology that is particularly valuable in relating intensive field work to emerging theory. By analyzing data according to its theoretical import as it is collected, the constant comparative method of qualitative analysis grounds the data in the emerging research process. The researcher alternates between theoretical implications and the collection of data, with the emerging theory guiding the continuing accumulation of data. This approach is particularly applicable to longitudinal studies. The emphasis is on generating rather than verifying theory. These methods are particularly useful for exploratory studies, such as that conducted within Victory Hospital.

NOTES

1. Barry G. Glaser and Anselm L. Strauss, The Discovery of Grounded Theory: Strategies for Qualitative Research (Chicago: Aldine, 1967).

2. Selwyn W. Becker and Thomas L. Whisler, "The Innovative Organization: A Selective View of Current Theory and Research," Journal of Business 40 (October 1967): 409.

3. Hans O. Mauksch, "Studying the Hospital," in Pathways to Data: Field Methods for Studying Ongoing Social Organizations, ed. Robert W. Habenstein (Chicago: Aldine, 1970), p. 192.

4. Wolf V. Heydebrand, Hospital Bureaucracy: A Comparative Study of Organizations (New York: Dunellen, 1973), p. xxv. See also Allan D. Bauerschmidt, "The Hospital as a Prototype Organization," Hospital Administration 15 (Spring 1970).

5. Glaser and Strauss, op. cit.

ADDITIONAL REFERENCES ON METHODOLOGY

Bakan, David. On Methods: Towards a Reconstruction of Psychological Investigation. San Francisco: Jossey-Bass, 1969.

Filstead, William J., ed. Qualitative Methodology First-Hand
Involvement with the Social World. Chicago: Markham, 1970.

✓ Flook, E. Evelyn, and Paul J. Sanazaro. Health Services Research
and R & D Perspective. Ann Arbor, Mich.: Health Administration Press, 1973.

Junker, Buford H. Field Work: An Introduction to the Social
Sciences. Chicago: University of Chicago Press, 1969.

McFarland, Dalton E. Research Methods in the Behavioral Sciences:
A Selected Bibliography. Monticello, Ill.: Council of Planning
Librarians, 1974.

O'Toole, Richard, ed. The Organization Management and Tactics
of Social Research. Cambridge, Mass.: Schenckman, 1971.

Stein, Franklin. Anatomy of Research in Allied Health. New York:
Wiley, 1976.

Wax, Rosalie. Doing Fieldwork: Warnings and Advice. Chicago:
University of Chicago Press, 1971.

MAJOR AREAS OF INVESTIGATION

Subject areas to be explored with informants.

1. Who are the key change agents in this hospital?
2. How well does the hospital define and solve its problems?
3. What are some examples of innovation or change within the last five years?
4. Do innovation and change produce stress in the organization? If so, where and how? What are the reactions to such stress?
5. What are the sources of any innovation or change?
   a. Leaders
   b. Outsiders
   c. Insiders
   d. Professional/technical sources
   e. Boundary spanners
   f. Consultants
   g. Research findings
6. Are some parts of the organization more successful in change and innovation than other parts?
7. Does resistance to change occur? In what form? Where? How is it dealt with?
8. Are changes and innovations forced or voluntary?
9. Have totally new structural forms appeared anywhere?
10. What management and organizational changes are made necessary by technical changes in medicine and health care?
11. What mechanisms are used to encourage and reward innovative behavior? That is, suggestion systems and so forth.
12. Is the overall climate or environment conducive to change and innovation?
13. What is the pattern by which an innovation or change is carried out?
    a. Planning
    b. Announcement
    c. Participation
    d. Diffusion
    e. Assessment, evaluation
    f. Staff services
14. Have any changes or innovations been scrapped or significantly changed due to their failure?

15. Are there any organizational myths or belief systems which discourage, impede, or prevent innovation and change?
16. How are proposals for change and innovation treated?
   a. Evaluation
   b. Testing
   c. Screening
   d. Diffusion
   e. Implementation

INTERVIEW PROTOCOL AND GENERAL AREAS PREPARED FOR FIELD INVESTIGATIONS OF MANAGERIAL INNOVATION AND CHANGE IN HOSPITALS

I. Interviewing Protocols
  A. Site
      1. Primary case study to be conducted at Victory Hospital, a unit of the Norfield Medical Complex
      2. Additional interviews with chief administrators in other hospitals in the same region as Victory Hospital
  B. Central Theme
      1. To explore with each informant the nature of innovation and change processes in the management and organization at Victory Hospital
      2. To explore the sources, nature, and organizational components of managerial innovation and change
      3. To examine the attitudes and involvement of the informants in the above processes
  C. Informants
      1. Initial informants will be selected after a preliminary study of the organization structure
      2. Key informants will be selected from the top administrative group
      3. Additional informants will be selected as the study progresses
      4. Key informants will be interviewed more than once
  D. Data Collection
      1. The main instrument for data collection is the unstructured interview, using open-ended questions
      2. Each initial interview will obtain a minimum amount of data through structured questions relating to informant, his position, experience, status, and so on
      3. Observation is an ancillary source of data, to be used mainly in connection with interviewing
  E. Interview Procedures
      1. Request interview appointment either in person or by telephone
      2. Time required, approximately 1 to 2 hours, each interview
      3. Recording equipment not used during interview. Note taking may be desirable but should be at a minimum

4. Following interview, interviewer will complete his rough notes and/or dictate full contents on recorder. Dictation should occur as soon as possible after interview. Try to achieve as close to a verbatim report as possible

5. Format of interview (general)
   a) Interviewer introduces himself and purpose
      (i) Build rapport
      (ii) Answer informant's questions
   b) State that all information provided will be kept absolutely confidential and used without identifying informant
   c) Obtain and record preliminary data (facts regarding: informant, position, personal data, and so on)
   d) Series of open-ended questions and follow-up probes
   e) Closure is important
      (i) Thank the informant
      (ii) Ask informant if you may see him again later on as the study progresses
   f) Developing interview content
      (i) With open-ended questions, try to get informant to converse about situations he has been involved in that show how innovation and change came about
      (ii) When attitudes or opinions are expressed, ask for examples and illustration, or concrete situations in which informant has knowledge or firsthand experience
      (iii) Get specific names, times, places, and so on, wherever possible. Ask for supporting documents or accept them if offered
      (iv) Let informant "run with the ball" whenever possible. Ask questions to get clarification, greater depth, and so on. Get a full account of each incident or area of discussion. Better to have few areas in depth than large number of shallow or incomplete areas
      (v) Let informant choose areas of importance or interest to him, but when he runs out of gas, be prepared to give him an assist to continue to the next area
      (vi) Rephrasing informant's comments can show your understanding, empathy, and so on, and encourage him to continue

        (vii) Interviewer should not give own opinions, attitudes, value judgments unless directly asked. Keep emotionally uninvolved, but interested in informant and his problems

II. Areas of Exploration

    A. We are primarily interested in innovation defined as "the introduction into an applied situation of means or ends that are new to that situation"

    B. Purely inventive, creative activity or new discoveries of a scientific or technical nature are rare. These are of interest and should be noted where found, but these will not be the sole or primary areas of study

        1. Technological, productive, or service changes will be of interest mainly on account of their effects in changing managerial or organizational practices

        2. Change or innovation in the following areas should be carefully explored with informants:

           a) Managerial behavior, expectations, or techniques

           b) Organization structure or design

           c) Policies, practices, or major decisions involving substantial change

           d) Changes in objectives, aims, purposes, goals

           e) Changes in work flow, technical equipment, work systems, task allocations, and so on

CODING PROTOCOLS

PROJECT ON INNOVATION AND CHANGE
IN HOSPITAL MANAGEMENT

Subject: Tentative listing of conceptual categories, definitions of categories, and properties of categories for coding and analysis of research data.

The following categories of data are suggested from study of interview materials to data:

1. Ideation
2. Change processes
3. Capabilities of people
4. Evaluation and assessment process
5. Adaption process
6. Diffusion-implementation
7. Role behaviors
8. Organizational framework

The eight categories and their properties are defined in the following lists.

Ideation

The discovery, formation, and proposing of ideas for change in the organization

Properties

1. Loci (origin) of ideas: high, medium, and lower levels of the organization
2. Forces evoking ideation: motives, pressures, needs, problems
3. Emotional-temperamental constraints: inertia, fear of criticism, feelings of futility, lack of success
4. Favorableness or unfavorableness of the organization climate for producing ideas

5. Open- versus closed-mindedness of administrators or officials
6. Quality of ideation: degree of originality, spontaneity, inventiveness, imagination
7. Presence or absence of "idea men," mavericks, geniuses
8. Presence or absence of idea-inducing reward structure

Change

The processes of growth, evolution, development, or adaptation

Properties

1. Degree of importance to the organization
2. Internal versus external forces for change
3. Planned versus unplanned change
4. Problem recognition and definition
5. Frequency, volume, and pace of change
6. Types or areas of change
7. Level of acceptance versus resistance to change
8. Operational strategies for achieving change

Capabilities of People

Characteristics of individuals in the organization who produce ideas and proposals for change or influence the effectiveness of change

Properties

1. Inquisitiveness
2. Resourcefulness
3. Pride or job satisfaction
4. Skills and knowledge
5. Insight
6. Professional attitudes
7. Persistence
8. Trust in others
9. Emotional properties—affect
10. Change-oriented values

Evaluation and Assessment Process

The process of judging potential risks, impact, or success and the continuing desirability of an idea, innovation, or change

Properties

1. Degree of persuasion (selling) needed
2. Use or nonuse of reference groups for technical or professional support
3. Planning, staff work, research required
4. Time spans: low, medium, high
5. Fairness of administrators who make decisions
6. Following channels of authority for getting approval
7. Measurement, appraisal procedures
8. Cost-benefit analysis
9. Choice and use of criteria

Adoption

The decision to try, adopt, use, or introduce into an applied situation means or ends that are new to that situation

Properties

1. Rate of adoption
2. Latitude, discretion for adoption
3. Locus (level) of final approval
4. Proportion of adoptions to ideas of proposals for change
5. Factors for rejection, delay
6. Adoption by administrative fiat against resistance
7. Handling of rejected ideas of proposals

Diffusion-Implementation

Manner in which an idea, change, or proposal is integrated into the organizational context and made operational

Properties

1. Impact of adoption in one unit on other, related parts of the organization
2. Extent to which predicted benefits actually occur

3. Degree of acceptance: tolerance, passive adoption, enthusiastic adoption
4. Communicating the decision to adopt or the new ideas, changes
5. Training and retraining of personnel
6. Failures (recidivism), return to previous way
7. Problems of coping, adjustment, adaptation, and fine tuning

Role Behaviors

Behavioral and performance expectations of others relative to a given set of task responsibilities

Properties

1. Change agents
2. Boundary spanner versus provincial
3. Reference group phenomena
4. Expectations
5. Group spirit
6. Role conflict

Organizational Framework

Structures, processes, and attributes of the organization that inhibit or facilitate creativity, innovation, and change

Properties

1. Degree of constraint: open versus closed system
2. Degree or level of trust
3. Impact of departments or other units on each other
4. Organizational philosophy
5. History and tradition
6. Disruption of physical environment
7. Disturbance of power relationships
8. Interdepartmental or other interunit conflict and coordination
9. Presence or absence of organization slack
10. Bureaucracy: need for rigidity, formality, routinization, conformity, efficiency, stability
11. Degree of decentralization and feedback
12. Conformity versus independence of organization members

SELECTED BIBLIOGRAPHY

BOOKS AND MONOGRAPHS

Ackoff, Russell L., and Fred E. Emery. On Purposeful Systems. Chicago: Aldine-Atherton, 1972.

Alford, Robert R. Health Care Politics: Ideological and Interest Group Barriers to Reform. Chicago: University of Chicago Press, 1975.

Argyris, Chris. Diagnosing Human Relations in Organizations: A Case Study of a Hospital. New Haven, Conn.: Yale University Labor and Management Center, 1956.

Arnold, Mary F., L. Vaughn Blankenship, and John M. Hess, eds. Administering Health Systems: Issues and Perspectives. Chicago: Aldine-Atherton, 1971.

Aron, Raymond. Progress and Disillusion: The Dialectic of Modern Society. New York: New American Library, 1969.

Ashley, Joan. Hospitals, Paternalism, and the Role of the Nurse. New York: Teachers College Press, 1976.

Barron, Frank. Creativity and Psychological Health: Origins of Personal Vitality and Creative Freedom. New York: D. Van Nostrand, 1963.

Basil, Douglas C., and Curtis W. Cook. The Management of Change. New York: McGraw-Hill, 1974.

Bauerschmidt, Alan D., and Richard W. Thrust. Forecasting Change in the Health Care Industry. Columbia: University of South Carolina Press, 1973.

Belasco, James A., and Harrison M. Trice. The Assessment of Change in Training and Therapy. New York: McGraw-Hill, 1969.

Bell, David. The Coming of the Post-Industrial Society. New York: Basic Books, 1973.

Bender, A. Douglas, et al. A Delphic Study of the Future of Medicine. Philadelphia: Research and Development Division, Smith, Kline and French Laboratories, 1969.

Bennis, Warren G. The Unconscious Conspiracy: Why Leaders Can't Lead. New York: AMACOM, 1976.

_____, ed. American Bureaucracy, 2nd ed. New Brunswick, N.J.: Transaction Books', 1972.

_____. Changing Organizations. New York: McGraw-Hill, 1966.

_____, Kenneth D. Benne, and Robert Chin, eds. The Planning of Change, 2nd ed. New York: Holt, Rinehart and Winston, 1969.

Bhola, Harbans Singh. The Configurational Theory of Innovation Diffusion. Columbus: Ohio State University, College of Education, 1965.

Bloom, Bernard L. Changing Patterns in Psychiatric Care. New York: Behavioral Publications, 1975.

Bloom, Samuel W. The Doctor and His Patient: A Sociological Interpretation. New York: Free Press, 1965.

Blum, Henrik L. Planning for Health: Development and Application of Social Change Theory. New York: Behavioral Publications, 1974.

Blumberg, M. S. Shared Services for Hospitals. Chicago: American Hospital Association, 1966.

Brinkers, Henry S., ed. Decision Making: Creativity, Judgment, and Systems. Columbus: Ohio State University Press, 1972.

Brodie, Donald C. The Challenge to Pharmacy in Times of Change. Washington, D.C.: American Pharmaceutical Association and American Society of Hospital Pharmacists, 1966.

Brown, Esther Lucille. Nursing Reconsidered: A Study of Change, parts 1 and 2. Philadelphia: Lippincott, 1971.

Brown, Montague, and Howard L. Lewis. Hospital Management Systems: Multi-Unit Organization and Delivery of Health Care. Germantown, Md.: Aspen Systems Corporation, 1976.

Burling, Temple, Edith M. Lentz, and Robert N. Wilson. The Give and Take in Hospitals: A Study of Human Organization in Hospitals. New York: Putnam's, 1956.

Burns, Eveline M. Health Services for Tomorrow: Trends and Issues. New York: Dunellen, 1973.

Carlson, Rick J. The End of Medicine. New York: Wiley, 1975.

Carter, Launor F. Knowledge Production and Utilization in Contemporary Organizations. Santa Monica, Calif.: Systems Development Corporation, 1968.

Caudill, William S. The Psychiatric Hospital as a Small Society. Cambridge, Mass.: Harvard University Press, 1968.

Clelland, Rod. The Human Side of Hospital Administration. Englewood Cliffs, N.J.: Prentice-Hall, 1974.

Cochrane, A. L. Effectiveness and Efficiency: Random Reflections on Health Services. London: Nuffield Provincial Hospitals Trust, 1972.

Coe, R. M., ed. Planned Change in the Hospital: Case Studies of Organizational Innovation. New York: Praeger, 1970.

_____, and A. F. Wilson. Sociology of Medicine. New York: McGraw-Hill, 1970.

Coleman, James S., et al. Medical Innovation: A Diffusion Study. Indianapolis: Bobbs-Merrill, 1966.

Collen, M. F., ed. Technology and Health Care Systems in the 1980's: Proceedings of a Conference, January 19-21, 1972, San Francisco, California. Washington, D.C.: U.S. Department of Health, Education, and Welfare, Health Services and Mental Health Administration, National Center for Health Services Research and Development, DHEW Publication No. (HSM) 73-3016, 1973.

De Bono, Edward. Lateral Thinking: Creativity Step by Step. New York: Harper & Row, 1972.

Demone, Harold, Jr., and Dwight Harshberger, eds. Handbook of Human Service Organizations. New York: Behavioral Publications, 1973.

Derzon, Robert. "Should the Role of Pharmacist Be Redefined?" In Challenge to Pharmacy in the 70's. Edited by Joe B. Graber and Donald Brodie. Springfield, Va.: National Technical Information Service, 1971.

Donabedian, Avedis. Aspects of Medical Care Administration. Cambridge, Mass.: Harvard University Press, 1973.

Drake, David. "The Hospital as a Public Utility." In Regulating the Hospital. A Report of the 1972 National Forum on Hospital and Health Affairs, Department of Health Administration. Durham, N.C.: Duke University Press, 1973.

Dyer, Frederick C., and John M. Dyer. Bureaucracy vs. Creativity. Coral Gables, Fla.: University of Miami Press, 1965.

Dykens, J. W., R. W. Hyde, L. H. Orzack, and R. H. York. Strategies of Mental Hospital Change. Boston: Massachusetts Department of Mental Health, 1964.

Ewell, Charles. Relationships between Program Innovation and Hospital Governance. Madison: University of Wisconsin Press, 1974.

✓ Fabun, Don. The Dynamics of Change. Englewood Cliffs, N.J.: Prentice-Hall, 1967.

✓ Fendrock, John J. Managing in Times of Radical Change. New York: American Management Association, 1971.

Fischer, E. F., Jr., and J. C. Sherick. Guidelines for Health Services Research and Development: Sharing, Centralization, and Consolidation of Laboratory and Diagnostic Services: Bibliography. Health Services Research Center of the Hospital Research and Education Trust and Northwestern University. KHEW Publication (HSM) 72-3036. Washington, D.C.: U.S. Government Printing Office, 1972.

Flook, E. Evelyn, and Paul J. Sanazaro, eds. Health Service Research and R & D Perspective. Ann Arbor: Health Administration Press, University of Michigan, 1974.

Forward Plan for Health. Washington, D.C.: U.S. Department of Health, Education, and Welfare, 1975.

Fottler, Myron D. Manpower Substitution in the Hospital Industry: A Study of New York City Voluntary and Municipal Hospital Systems. New York: Praeger, 1972.

Freidson, Eliot. Profession of Medicine: A Study of the Sociology of Applied Knowledge. New York: Dodd, Mead, 1970.

_____. Professional Dominance: The Social Structure of Medical Care. Chicago: Aldine, 1970.

_____, ed. The Hospital in Modern Society. New York: Free Press, 1963.

_____, and Judith Lorber, eds. Medical Men and Their Work: A Sociological Reader. Chicago: Aldine-Atherton, 1971.

Gardner, John W. Self-Renewal: The Individual and the Innovative Society. New York: Harper & Row, 1964.

Geiger, J. "The New Doctor." In The New Professionals. Edited by Ronald Gross and Paul Osterman. New York: Simon & Schuster, 1972.

Georgopoulos, Basil S. Hospital Organization Research: Review and Sourcebook. Philadelphia: Saunders, 1975.

_____. "The Hospital as an Organization and Problem Solving System." In Organization Research on Health Institutions. Edited by Basil S. Georgopoulos. Ann Arbor: Institute for Social Research, University of Michigan, 1972.

Gilb, Corinne Lathrop. Hidden Hierarchies: The Professions and Government. New York: Harper & Row, 1966.

Glaser, W. A. Social Settings and Medical Organizations: A Cross-National Study of the Hospitals. Chicago: Aldine-Atherton, 1973.

Golladay, Frederick, and Kenneth Smith. Regulating the Health Industry: A Study Prepared for the Health Planning Council. Madison: Wisconsin Regional Medical Program, 1974.

Goss, Mary E. W. "Patterns of Bureaucracy among Staff Physicians." In The Hospital in Modern Society. Edited by Eliot Freidson. New York: Free Press, 1963.

_____. "Physicians in Bureaucracy: A Case Study of Professional Pressures on Organizational Roles." Ph.D. diss., Columbia University, 1959.

Green, John, Raymond Moss, and Colon Jackson. Hospital Research Briefing Problems. London: King Edward's Hospital Fund for London, 1971.

Green, Stephen. The Hospital: An Organizational Analysis. London: Blackie and Son, 1974.

Greenblatt, Milton, Myron Sharaf, and Evelyn M. Stone. Dynamics of Institutional Change: The Hospital in Transition. Pittsburgh: University of Pittsburgh Press, 1971.

Greenfield, Harry I. Hospital Efficiency and Public Policy. New York: Praeger, 1973.

Griffith, John R., Lewis D. Weeks, and James H. Sullivan. The McPherson Experiment: Expanded Community Hospital Services. Ann Arbor, Mich.: Cooperative Information Center for Hospital Management Studies, 1967.

Guest, Robert. "The Role of the Doctor in Institutional Management." In Organization Research on Health Institutions. Edited by Basil Georgopoulos. Ann Arbor: University of Michigan, 1972.

Hage, Jerald, and Michael Aiken. Social Change in Complex Organizations. New York: Random House, 1970.

Hasenfeld, Yeheskel, and Richard A. English, eds. Human Service Organizations: Book of Readings. Ann Arbor: University of Michigan Press, 1974.

Havelock, Ronald G. Planning for Innovation through Dissemination and Utilization of Knowledge. Ann Arbor: Institute for Social Research, University of Michigan, 1969.

_____, et al. Training for Change Agents: A Guide to the Design of Training Programs in Education and Other Fields. Ann Arbor: Center for Research on Utilization of Scientific Knowledge, University of Michigan, 1973.

_____. Bibliography on Knowledge Utilization and Dissemination. Rev. ed. Ann Arbor: Center for Research on Utilization of Scientific Knowledge, Institution for Social Research, University of Michigan, 1972.

Hepner, James O., and Donna M. Hepner. The Health Strategy Game: A Challenge for Reorganization and Management. Ch. 8, "Innovations on Health Care System." St. Louis, Mo.: Mosby, 1973.

Heydebrand, Wolf V. Hospital Bureaucracy: A Comparative Study of Organizations. New York: Dunellen, 1973.

Hirschfield, Daniel S. The Lost Reform. Cambridge, Mass.: Harvard University Press, 1970.

Hodgson, Richard C., Daniel J. Levinson, and Abraham Zaleznik. The Executive Role Constellation: An Analysis of Personality and Role Relations in Management. Boston: Harvard University Division of Research, Graduate School of Business Administration, 1965.

Hoffer, Eric. The Ordeal of Change. New York: Harper & Row, 1963.

Hughes, Everett C. Men and Their Work. New York: Free Press, 1958.

Huse, Edgar F. Organization Development and Change. St. Paul, Minn.: West Publishing Co., 1975.

Illich, Ivan. Medical Nemesis: The Expropriation of Health. London: Calder and Boyars, 1975.

_____. Tools for Conviviality. New York: Harper & Row, 1973.

Jaeger, B. Jon, ed. A Decade of Implementation: The Multiple Management Concept Revisited. Durham, N.C.: Department of Health Administration, Duke University, 1975.

Jaques, Elliott. Work, Creativity, and Social Justice. New York: International University Press, 1970.

Jelinek, Richard. An Organizational Approach to Improved Patient Care. Battle Creek, Mich.: W. K. Kellogg Foundation, 1971.

Johns, Edward A. The Sociology of Organizational Care. Oxford, New York: Pergamon Press, 1974.

Kaluzny, Arnold D., J. T. Gentry, and J. E. Veney, eds. Innovation in Health Care Organizations. Chapel Hill: School of Public Health, University of North Carolina, 1974.

Kaufman, Herbert. The Limits of Organizational Change. University: University of Alabama Press, 1971.

Kneller, George F. The Art and Science of Creativity. New York: Holt, Rinehart and Winston, 1965.

Knutson, A. L. The Individual, Society, and Health Behavior. New York: Russell Sage Foundation, 1965.

Koestler, Arthur. The Act of Creation. New York: Macmillan, 1964.

Kovner, Anthony R. "The Hospital Administrator and Organization Effectiveness." In Organization Research on Health Institutions. Edited by Basil Georgopoulos. Ann Arbor: Institute for Social Research, University of Michigan, 1972.

Lasswell, Harold D. "The Social Setting of Creativity." In Creativity in Its Cultivation. Edited by Harold Anderson. New York: Harper & Row, 1959.

Leavitt, Harold J. "Applied Organizational Change in Industry." In Handbook of Organization. Edited by J. G. March. Chicago: Rand McNally, 1965.

Levey, Samuel, and N. Paul Loomba. Health Care Administration: A Managerial Perspective. Philadelphia: Lippincott, 1973.

Lippitt, Ronald. "The Use of Social Research to Improve Social Practice." In Concepts for Social Change. Baltimore: National Training Laboratory, 1967.

_____, Jeanne Watson, and Bruce Westley. The Dynamics of Planned Change. New York: Harcourt, Brace, 1958.

Luck, R. M., J. Luckman, V.W. Smith, and J. Stinger. Patients, Hospitals, and Operational Research. London: Tavistock Publications, 1971.

McGraw, Richard M. Ferment in Medicine. Philadelphia: Saunders Co., 1966.

McLaughlin, Curtis P., and Alan Sheldon. The Future and Medical Care. Cambridge, Mass.: Ballinger, 1974.

Mann, Floyd C. "Studying and Creating Change: A Means to Understanding Social Organization." In Industrial Relations Research Association: Research in Industrial Human Relations: A Critical Appraisal, by C. M. Arensberg. New York: Harper & Row, 1957.

Marram, Gwen, et al. Cost-Effectiveness of Primary Team Nursing. Wakefield, Mass.: Contemporary Publishing, 1976.

Mason, Robert. "An Ordinal Scale for Measuring the Adoption Process." In Studies of Innovation and of Communications to the Public. Edited by E. Katz et al. Stanford, Calif.: Stanford University Institute for Communication Research, 1962.

Mauksch, Hans O. "Nursing: Churning for Change." In Handbook of Medical Sociology, 2nd ed. Edited by Howard Freeman, Sol Levine, and Leo G. Reeder. Englewood Cliffs, N.J.: Prentice-Hall, 1972.

May, Rollo. The Courage to Create. New York: Norton, 1975.

Mechanic, David. The Growth of Bureaucratic Medicine: An Inquiry into the Dynamics of Patient Behavior and the Organization of Medical Care. New York: Wiley, 1976.

_____. Patient Behavior and the Organization of Medical Care, Research and Analytic Report Series. Madison, Wis.: Center for Medical Sociology and Health Services Research, 1973.

_____. Public Expectations in Health Care: Essays on the Changing Organization of Health Services. New York: Wiley, 1972.

_____, et al. The Growth of Bureaucratic Medicine. New York: Wiley, 1976.

Mendelsohn, Everett, Judith P. Swazey, and Irene Traviss, eds. Human Aspects of Biomedical Innovation. Cambridge, Mass.: Harvard University Press, 1971.

Metzger, Norman. Personnel Administration in Health Services Industries. New York: Spectrum Publications, 1975.

Moos, Rudolf H. Evaluating Treatment Environments: A Social-Ecological Approach. New York: Wiley, 1974.

Neuhauser, Duncan. The Relationships between Administrative Activities and Hospital Performance. Chicago: University of Chicago Center for Health Administration Studies, 1971.

Pelz, Donald C. "Conditions for Innovation." In Organization Theory: A Behavioral Approach. Edited by Walter A. Hill and Douglas Egan. Boston: Allyn and Bacon, 1966.

Perrow, Charles. "Goals and Power Structure: A Historical Case Study." In The Hospital in Modern Society. Edited by Eliot Freidson. New York: Free Press, 1963.

Pressman, Jeffrey L., and Aaron Wildavsky. Implementation. Berkeley: University of California Press, 1974.

Prince, George M. The Practice of Creativity: A Manual for Dynamic Group Problem Solving. New York: Harper & Row, 1970.

Rakich, Jonathan S., Beaufort B. Longest, Jr., and Thomas R. O'Donovan. Managing Health Care Organizations. Philadelphia: Saunders, 1977.

Reissman, Leonard, and John H. Roher, eds. Change and Dilemmas in the Nursing Profession. New York: Putnam's, 1957.

Roemer, Milton I., and Jay W. Friedman. Doctors in Hospitals: Medical Staff Organization and Hospital Performance. Baltimore: Johns Hopkins Press, 1971.

Rogers, Everett M. Communication of Innovation. 2nd ed. New York: Free Press, 1971.

Rosenfeld, L. S. Ambulatory Care: Planning and Organization. Report no. PB-204-925. Springfield, Va.: National Technical Information Service, U.S. Department of Commerce, 1971.

Rosner, Stanley, and Lawrence E. Abt. The Creative Expression. St. Cloud, Minn.: North Star Press, 1975.

Rosow, Jerome M., ed. The Worker and the Job: Coping with Change. Englewood Cliffs, N.J.: Prentice-Hall, 1974.

Rossi, Jean J., and William J. Filstead, eds. The Therapeutic Community: A Source Book. New York: Behavioral Publications, 1973.

Rowbottom, Ralph, et al. Hospital Organization. New York: Crane-Russak, 1973.

Rowe, Lloyd A., and William B. Boise, eds. Organizational and Managerial Innovation: A Reader. Pacific Palisades, Calif.: Goodyear Publishing Co., 1973.

Rutstein, David D. The Coming Revolution in Medicine. Cambridge, Mass.: MIT Press, 1967.

Schein, Edgar H., and Warren G. Bennis. Personal and Organizational Change through Group Methods. New York: Wiley, 1965.

Schon, Donald A. Technology and Change. New York: Delacorte Press, 1967.

Schulberg, Herbert C., Alan Sheldon, and Frank Baker, eds. Program Evaluation in the Health Fields. New York: Behavioral Publications, 1970.

Schulman, Jay. Remaking an Organization: Innovation in a Specialized Psychiatric Hospital. Albany: State University of New York Press, 1969.

Schwartz, Harry. The Case for American Medicine. New York: David McKay, 1973.

Sheldon, Alan. Organizational Issues in Health Care Management. New York: Spectrum Publications, 1975.

Smith, David B., and Arnold D. Kaluzny. The White Labyrinth: Understanding the Organization of Health Care. Berkeley, Calif: McCutchan Publishing Corporation, 1975.

Somers, Anne R. Health Care in Transition: Directions for the Future. Chicago: Hospital Research and Educational Trust, 1971.

_____. Hospital Regulation: The Dilemma of Public Policy. Princeton, N.J.: Industrial Relations Section, Princeton University, 1969.

Starkweather, David, Louis Gelwicks, and Robert Newcomes. Delphi Forecasting of Health Care Organizations, Paper no. 1. Berkeley: School of Public Health, University of California, 1973.

Stein, Morris I. Stimulating Creativity, vol. I. New York: Academic Press, 1974.

Strauss, Ansel. "The Structure and Ideology of American Nursing: An Interpretation." In The Nursing Profession. Edited by F. David. New York: Wiley, 1966.

Strauss, Robert. "Hospital Organization from the Viewpoint of Patient-Centered Goals." In Organization Research on Health Institutions. Edited by Basil Georgopoulos. Ann Arbor: Institute for Social Research, University of Michigan, 1972.

Taves, Marvin, Ronald G. Cronin, and James Eugene Haas. Role Conception, Vocational Success, and Satisfaction: A Study of Student and Professional Nurses. Columbus: Ohio State University Press, 1963.

Taylor, James C. Technology and Planned Organizational Change. Ann Arbor: Institute for Social Research, University of Michigan, 1971.

Thompson, Victor A. Bureaucracy and Innovation. University: University of Alabama Press, 1060.

Toomey, Robert E. "Governance of the Hospital, Place of the Trustee." In The Governance of Hospitals, A Report of the 1970 National Forum on Hospital and Health Affairs. Durham, N.C.: Duke University Graduate Program in Hospital Administration, 1970.

Tushman, Michael. Organizational Change: An Exploratory Study and Case History. Ithaca, N.Y.: New York State School of Industrial and Labor Relations, Cornell University, 1974.

U.S. Department of Health, Education, and Welfare, U.S. Public Health Service, Division of Community Health Services, American Public Health Association, eds. Medical Care in Transition, vol. I, 1949-1957; vol. IV, 1967. Washington, D.C.: U.S. Government Printing Office.

Warner, Aaron W., Dean Morse, and Thomas E. Cooney, eds. The Environment of Change. New York: Columbia University Press, 1969.

Weissman, Harold H. Overcoming Mismanagement in the Human Service Professions: A Casebook of Staff Initiatives. San Francisco: Jossey-Bass, 1973.

White, Rodney F. "The Hospital Administrator's Emerging Professional Role." In Administering Health Systems: Issues and Perspectives. Chicago: Aldine-Atherton, 1971.

Wieland, George F., and Robert A. Ullrich. Organizations: Behavior, Design and Change. Homewood, Ill.: Richard D. Irwin, 1976.

Williams, Lawrence K. Managing Change: A Test of the Administration. Reprint Series no. 239. Ithaca, N.Y.: Cornell University, New York State School of Industrial and Labor Relations, 1968.

Wilson, James Q. "Innovation in Organization: Notes toward a Theory." In Approaches to Organizational Design. Edited by James D. Thompson. Pittsburgh: University of Pittsburgh Press, 1966.

Zald, Mayer N. "The Social Control of General Hospitals." In Organization Research on Health Institutions. Edited by Basil Georgopoulos. Ann Arbor: Institute for Social Research, University of Michigan, 1972.

Zaltman, Gerald, Robert Duncan, and Johnny Holbek. Innovation and Organizations. New York: Wiley, 1973.

Zander, Alvin F., Arthur R. Cohen, and Ezra Stotland. "Power and the Relations among Professions." In Studies in Social Power. Edited by D. Cartwright. Pp. 15-34. Ann Arbor: University of Michigan, 1959.

_____, _____, and _____. Role Relations in the Mental Health Professions. Ann Arbor: Institute for Social Research, University of Michigan, 1957.

ARTICLES

Aiken, Michael, and Jerald Hage. "Program Change and Organizational Properties: A Comparative Analysis." American Journal of Sociology 72 (March 1967): 503-19. Reprinted in Hasenfeld and English, Human Service Organizations.

Ainsworth, Thomas H., Jr. "The Physician as a Manager." Hospitals 44 (December 16, 1970): 53-55.

Alexander, T., W. Money, and T. Beatzoglou. "Multihospital Systems May Offer Solutions to Delivery Problems." Hospitals 50 (November 1, 1976): 73-76.

Armenakis, Achilles A., and Hubert S. Field. "Evaluation of Organizational Change Using Nonindependent Criterion Measures." Personnel Psychology 28 (Spring 1975): 39-44.

Austin, Charles J. "Emerging Roles and Responsibilities in Health Administration." In Education for Health Administration, vol. I. Report of the Commission on Education for Health Administration. Ann Arbor, Mich.: Health Administration Press, 1975.

_____. "What Is Health Administration?" Hospital Administration 19 (Summer 1974): 14-29.

Baker, Frank. "An Open Systems Approach to the Study of Mental Hospitals in Transition." Community Mental Health Journal 5 (October 1969): 403-12.

Beal, G. M., Everett M. Rogers, and J. M. Bohlon. "Validity of the Concept of Stages in the Adoption Process." Rural Sociology 22 (June 1957): 166-68.

Becker, M. "Sociometric Location and Innovativeness: Reformulation and Extension of the Diffusion Model." American Sociological Review 35 (April 1970): 267-82.

Bellin, Lowell E. "The Health Administrator as a Status Seeker." Journal of Medical Education 48 (October 1973): 896-904.

Ben-David, Joseph. "Roles and Innovations in Medicine." American Journal of Sociology 65 (May 1960): 557-68.

Benedict, B., et al. "The Clinical Experimental Approach to Assessing Organizational Change Efforts." Journal of Applied Behavioral Science 3 (July–August–September 1967): 347-80.

Bennis, Warren G. "Theory and Method in Applying Behavioral Science to Planned Organizational Change." Journal of Applied Behavioral Science 1 (October-November-December 1965): 337-60.

Blasingame, F. J. L. "Governance of Hospitals: The Case for Physicians as Board Members." Trustee 23 (September 1970): 21-25.

Bloomberg, Sanford. "Problems Associated with the Introduction of a Psychiatric Unit into a Rural General Hospital." American Journal of Psychiatry 130 (January 1973): 28-31.

Borman, L. D. "The Marginal Route of a Mental Hospital Innovation." Human Organization 29 (Spring 1970): 63-69.

Coles, A. B. "Role Articulation Needed among Health Care Providers." Urban Health 3 (April 1974): 46-63.

Diamant, A. "Innovation in Bureaucratic Institutions." Public Administration Review 27 (March 1967): 77-87.

Dickson, John W., and Dennis P. Slevin. "The Use of Semantic Differential Scales in Studying the Innovation Boundary." Academy of Management Journal 18 (June 1975): 381-88.

Downs, George W., and Lawrence B. Mohr. "Conceptual Issues in the Study of Innovation." Administrative Science Quarterly 21 (December 1976): 700-14.

Duncan, W. Jack. "The Knowledge Utilization Process in Management and Organization." Academy of Management Journal 15 (September 1972): 273-88.

Eitzen, D. S., and Norman R. Yetman. "Managerial Change, Longevity, and Organizational Effectiveness." Administrative Science Quarterly 17 (March 1973): 110-16.

Emery, John T., Robert J. Halonen, and Robin E. MacStravic. "The Prediction and Planning of Organizational Change in Health Care Institutions." Journal of Economics and Business 28 (Spring/Summer 1976): 242-48.

Ferber, Bernard. "An Analysis of Chain-operated For-Profit Hospitals." Health Services Research 6 (Spring 1971): 49-60.

Fink, Stephen L., Joel Beak, and Kenneth Taddeo. "Organizational Crisis and Change." Journal of Applied Behavioral Science 7 (January/February 1971): 15-37.

Gerstenfeld, A. "Interdependence and Innovation." Omega 5, no. 1 (1977): 35-42.

Goldberg, Theodore, and Ronald Hemmelgarn. "Who Governs the Hospitals?" Hospitals 45 (August 1, 1971): 72-79.

Goods, William J. "Encroachment, Charlatanism and the Emerging Profession: Psychology, Sociology, and Medicine." American Sociological Review 25 (December 1960): 902-14.

Goss, Mary E. W. "Organizational Goals and Quality of Medical Care: Evidence from Comparative Research on Hospitals." Journal of Health and Social Behavior 2 (December 1970): 255-68.

Greenfield, T. Barri. "Organizations as Social Inventions: Rethinking Assumptions about Change." Journal of Applied Behavioral Science 9 (September-October 1973): 551-74.

Greiner, Larry E. "Antecedents of Planned Organizational Change." Journal of Applied Behavioral Science 3 (January-March 1967): 51-85.

Gruenfeld, Leopold, and Saleem Kassum. "Supervisory Style and Organizational Effectiveness in a Pediatric Hospital." Personnel Psychology 26 (Winter 1973): 531-44.

Hage, Jerald, and Michael Aiken. "Program Change and Organizational Properties: A Comparative Analysis." American Journal of Sociology 72 (March 1967): 503-19.

Hage, Jerald, and J. Dewar. "The Prediction of Organizational Performance: The Case of Program Innovation." Administrative Science Quarterly 18 (September 1973): 279-90.

Hasenfeld, Yeheskel. "People Processing Organizations: An Exchange Approach." American Sociological Review 37 (June 1972): 256-63.

Hickey, W. J. "The Functions of the Hospital Board of Directors." Hospital Administration 17 (Summer 1972): 43-53.

Hughes, Everett C. "Professions." Daedalus 94 (Fall 1963): 655-69.

Junghare, Y. N., and Roy Prodipto. "The Relations of Health-Practice Innovations to Social Background Characteristics and Attitudes." Rural Sociology 28 (December 1963): 394-400.

Kaluzny, Arnold D. "Innovations in Health Services: Theoretical Framework and Review of Research." Health Services Research 9 (Summer 1974): 101-20.

_____, and James E. Veney. "Who Influences Decisions in the Hospital? Not Even the Administrator Really Knows." Modern Hospital 119 (December 1972): 52-53.

_____, _____, and John T. Gentry. "Innovation of Health Services: A Comparative Study of Hospitals and Health Departments." Health and Society 52 (Winter 1974): 51-82.

Katz, Elihu, Martin L. Levin, and H. Hamilton. "Traditions of Research on the Diffusion of Innovation." American Sociological Review 28 (April 1963): 237-52.

King, Albert S. "Expectation Effects in Organizational Change." Administrative Science Quarterly 19 (June 1974): 221-30.

Kirton, M. J., and Glenn Mulligan. "Correlates of Managers' Attitudes toward Change." Journal of Applied Psychology 58 (August 1973): 101-07.

Knight, Kenneth E. "A Descriptive Model of the Intra-Firm Innovation Process." Journal of Business 40 (October 1967): 478-96.

Kovner, Anthony R. "Governing Boards." Hospital Administration 20 (Winter 1975): 65-72.

Kralewski, John Edward. "Leadership in the Evolving Health System." Hospital Administration 16 (Spring 1971): 7-14.

Lave, J. R., L. B. Lave, and T. E. Morton. "The Physician's Assistant: Exploration of the Concept." Hospitals 45 (June 2, 1971): 42-51.

Lawrence, Paul R. "How to Deal with Resistance to Change." Harvard Business Review 32 (May/June 1954): 49-57.

Levenstein, A. "Effective Change Agents." Hospitals 50 (December 16, 1976): 71-74.

Lindemann, Eric. "Social System Factors as Determinants of Resistance to Change." American Journal of Orthopsychiatry 35 (April 1965): 544-57.

Little, Delores. "The Nurse Specialist." American Journal of Nursing 67 (March 1967): 552-56.

Loy, John W., Jr. "Social Psychological Characteristics of Innovators." American Sociological Review 34 (February 1969): 73-82.

Lynton, Rolf P. "Linking an Innovative Subsystem into the System." Administrative Science Quarterly 14 (December 1969): 398-416.

Lyon, Herbert L., and John M. Ivancevich. "An Exploratory Investigation of Organizational Climate and Job Satisfaction in a Hospital." Academy of Management Journal 17 (December 1974): 635-48.

Lystad, Mary H. "Institutional Planning for Social Change." Sociology and Social Research 44 (January/February 1959): 156-71.

Marmor, Judd, Viola W. Bernard, and Perry Ottenborg. "Psychodynamics of Group Opposition to Health Programs." American Journal of Orthopsychiatry 30 (April 1960): 330-45.

Mechanic, David. "The Power to Resist Change among Low-Ranking Personnel." Personnel Administration 26 (July/August 1963): 5-11.

Menzel, Herbert. "Innovation, Integration, and Marginality: A Survey of Physicians." American Sociological Review 25 (October 1960): 704-13.

_____, and Elihu Katz. "Social Relations and Innovation in the Medical Professions." Public Opinion Quarterly 19 (Winter 1955-56): 337-52.

Moore, T. F., and B. E. Lorimer. "The Matrix Organization in Business and Health Care Institutions: A Comparison." Hospital and Health Services Administration 21 (Fall 1976): 26-34.

Neuhauser, Duncan. "The Hospital as a Matrix Organization." Hospital Administration 17 (Fall 1972): 8-25.

Pearlin, Leonard I. "Sources of Resistance to Change in a Mental Hospital." American Journal of Sociology 68 (November 1962): 325-34.

Perry, Astor, Gene A. Sullivan, Robert J. Dolan, and C. Paul March. "The Adoption Process: 'S' Curve or 'J' Curve?" Rural Sociology 32 (June 1967): 220-22.

Pfeffer, Jeffrey. "Size, Composition, and Function of Hospital Boards of Directors: A Study of Organization Environment Linkage." Administrative Science Quarterly 18 (September 1973): 349-64.

Pierce, Jon L., and Andre L. Delbecq. "Organization Structure, Individual Attitudes, and Innovation." Academy of Management Review 2 (January 1977): 27-37.

Platou, Carl N., and James A. Rice. "Multihospital Holding Companies." Harvard Business Review 50 (May/June 1972): 14-21, 146.

Price, James L. "Use of New Knowledge in Organizations." Human Organization 23 (Fall 1964): 224-34.

Putney, Snell, and Gladys J. Putney. "Radical Innovation and Prestige." American Sociological Review 27 (August 1962): 548-51.

Regenstreif, Donna I. "Innovation in Hospital-Based Ambulatory Care: Some Sources, Patterns, and Implications of Change." Human Organization 36 (Spring 1977): 43-49.

Revans, Reginald W. "Research into Hospital Management and Organization." Health and Society 44 (July 1966): 3.

Robins, A. J. "Governing Boards and Decision Making." Administration in Mental Health 4 (Fall/Winter 1976): 19-25.

Ronco, Paul G. "Human Factors Applied to Hospital Patient Care." Human Factors 14 (October 1972): 461-70.

Rosner, Martha. "Administrative Controls and Innovation." Behavioral Science 13 (January 1968): 36-43.

Rothwell, R. J., et al. "Some Methodological Aspects of Innovation Research." Omega 5, no. 4 (1977).

Rubenstein, Albert H. "Behavioral Factors Influencing the Adoption of an Experimental Information System by Medical Researchers and Clinicians in Six Hospitals." Catalog of Selected Documents in Psychology 2 (Summer 1972): 101-02.

Rushing, William. "Differences in Profit and Non-Profit Organizations: A Study of Effectiveness and Efficiency in General Short-Stay Hospitals." Administrative Science Quarterly 19 (December 1974): 474-85.

Sapolsky, Harvey M. "Organizational Structure and Innovation." Journal of Business 40 (October 1967): 497-510.

Sayles, L. R. "The Innovation Process: An Organizational Analysis." Journal of Management Studies 11 (October 1974): 190-204.

Schulz, Rockwell, and Alton C. Johnson. "Conflict in Hospitals." Hospital Administration 16 (Summer 1971): 36-50.

Scott, W. Richard. "Some Implications of Organization Theory Research on Health Services," part 2. Health and Society 44 (October 1966): 35-59.

Seashore, Stanley E., and David G. Bowers. "Durability of Organizational Change." American Psychologist 25 (March 1970): 227-33.

Seide, Marilyn, and Carol J. Eagle. "Hospital Confrontation: A Cry for Help and Technique for Change." American Journal of Orthopsychiatry 43 (January 1973): 79-85.

Slevin, Dennis P. "The Innovation Boundary: A Replication with Increased Cost." Administrative Science Quarterly 18 (March 1973): 71-75.

_____. "The Innovation Boundary: A Specific Model and Some Empirical Results." Administrative Science Quarterly 4 (December 1971): 515-31.

Starkweather, David B. "The Rationale for Decentralization in Large Hospitals." Hospital Administration 15 (Spring 1970): 27-45.

Stone, Thomas H. "Effects of Mode of Organization and Feedback Level on Creative Task Groups." Journal of Applied Psychology 55 (August 1971): 324-30.

Stull, R. J. "Many Concepts Mold Multi-Institutional Systems." Hospitals 51 (March 1977): 43-45.

Thompson, Victor A. "How Scientific Management Thwarts Innovation." Trans-Action 5 (June 1968): 51-55.

Tichy, Noel M. "Agents of Planned Social Change: Congruence of Values, Cognitions and Actions." Administrative Science Quarterly 19 (June 1974): 164-82.

Vance, Stanley C. "Administrators on Hospital Governing Boards: A Growing Trend." Trustee 26 (January 1973): 20-26.

Varnum, James W. "Administrator's View of Unit Dose Drug Distribution System." Canadian Journal of Hospital Pharmacy 26 (January/February 1973): 13-16.

Veney, James E., and Jahangir Khan. "Causal Paths in Elaboration of Organizational Structure: A Case of Hospital Services." Health Services Research 8 (Summer 1973): 139-50.

Veney, J. E., A. D. Kaluzny, J. R. Gentry, J. B. Sprague, and D. P. Duncan. "Implementation of Health Programs in Hospitals." Health Services Research 6 (Winter 1971): 350-62.

Walton, Richard E. "Successful Strategies for Diffusing Work Innovations." Journal of Contemporary Business 6 (Spring 1977): 1-22.

Weir, Mary, and Stephen Mills. "The Supervisor as a Change Catalyst." Industrial Relations Journal 4 (Winter 1973-74): 61-69.

Wiesbord, Marvin R. "Why Organization Development Hasn't Worked (So Far) in Medical Center." HCM Review 1 (Spring 1976): 17-28.

Wren, George R., and Sharon M. Hilgers. "Titles of Hospital Administrators." Hospital Administration 19 (Spring 1974): 68-82.

Zand, Dale E. "Collateral Organization: A New Change Strategy." Journal of Applied Behavioral Science 10 (January 1974): 63-89.

NAME INDEX

SUBJECT INDEX

admitting, 141-42, 189-92, 194-95, 250-51, 252
adoption, 131-55, 156-80 (see also diffusion)
assessment (see evaluation)
attitudes, 93-99, 175-77, 193-94
authority, 62 (see also delegation)

biomedical maintenance program, 184-87
board of trustees, 34-35, 56
boundary spanning, 121-30
bureaucracy, 43-45, 91-92, 156-80, 199, 259-63, 266-67

centralization, 62-81
change, 3-11, 45-50, 71-75, 131-55, 156-76, 209-18, 226-58, 263-65; agents of, 198-224; definitions of, 4-5; and delegation, 71-81; models of, 7-11, 132; and persuasion, 163-70; rejection of, 172-80; resistance to, 209-18, 226-58; slowing of, 36-39; technological, 263-65; theories of, 3
change agents, 199-224
computerization (see data processing)
conflict, 53-55, 126, 127, 162-63, 207-9; interdepartmental, 53-55
consultants, 121-23, 169
control, 64-65, 90-93, 106-8, 120-21, 124-26, 136-37; of ideation, 120-21; of manpower, 106-8
coordination, 55-56, 71, 170

creativity, 82-89, 99-104, 126-27, 276-77 (see also ideation)

data processing, 51-52, 139-42, 189-92, 229, 246-47
decentralization, 62-81; and delegation, 71-78
delegation, 71-78; in nursing, 75-78
diffusion, 5-6, 181-96, 187-92 (see also adoption)

environment, 45-46, 83-89, 120-29, 131, 137-39
evaluation of ideas, 156-80, 182-83
expectations, 110-30, 134-35

feedback model, 8, 12

goals (see planning)

health care, general, 1, 2-3, 6; change and, 3; innovation in, 6-7; organizations and, 1-2; research in, 6; system of, 1-2
health maintenance organizations, 202
hierarchy, organizational, 23, 89-90, 161-62, 200-4
hospital administration, 34-35, 47-50, 55-56, 64-65, 71-81, 199-204, 215, 259-77
hospitals, 2-3, 4-5, 6-7, 45-47, 64, 199-200, 226-27; and change, 4-5, 45-47, 226-27; innovation research in, 6-8
human relations (see interpersonal relations

ABOUT THE AUTHOR

DALTON E. McFARLAND, University Professor and Professor of Business Administration at the University of Alabama in Birmingham, is an internationally recognized authority in the fields of management, organization behavior, personnel management, and health care research.

Professor McFarland received his Ph.D. degree from Cornell University in 1952. He is the author of over 30 articles in scholarly and popular journals, numerous research monographs, and the editor, author, or co-author of several books, including a widely used text, Management: Foundations and Practices, 5th ed. (Macmillan, 1979). His most recent work deals with the concept of power in the field of nursing, published in Nursing Dimensions and in the Journal of Nursing Administration.

RAHMAN
DUNCAN
HOLBECK

Agreement — G arrange to meet need ...
What is needed is a PROACTIVE STRATEGY

PP 268   AIDS
             Drugs
             Alcohol Abuse. Etc
             Glue Sniff.